brain

CONNECTING
through COMPASSION

Cover design: DeHart and Company

Author Photography by: Bob Boyd
Interior Photography by: Joni James Aldrich
Cancer awareness ribbon and artwork: Anna Trenary at Creative Techniques

ISBN: 1451523858
ISBN-13: 9781451523850
LCCN: 2010904615

Printed in the United States of America

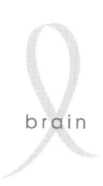

brain

CONNECTING
through COMPASSION:

Guidance for Family and Friends
of a Brain Cancer Patient

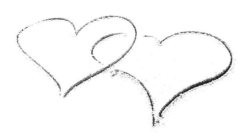

Joni James Aldrich

"I needed this book while caring for my brother Brian. The information has been carefully collected and delivered in a thoughtful way, and will benefit others as they fight to protect, assist and care for a brain cancer patient. You offer experience and empathy that is so desperately needed by those who cannot face another day of pain both before and after the loss of a loved one. Although I lost Brian, your writing has given me comfort and helped me to remember our cherished moments. This is one of the most relevant books I've read in a very long time."

Cynthia McKay, JD, MA

"Caring for someone with cancer is a labor of love, but it's so much more daunting when it involves the often inevitable changes associated with brain involvement. What Joni and Neysa have written is a compassionate and comprehensive guide that not only explains the changes that occur in patients with brain cancer, but also provides personal and pertinent information for their caregivers on how best to deal with those changes. As an advocate for cancer patients and their families—including those battling primary or secondary brain cancer—this book is an invaluable resource, and I highly recommend it."

Barbara L. Prisco, RN, OCN, MA, JD
Patient Advocate and Navigator

"I like this book because it's informative, heartfelt, and exceedingly practical."

William "Ben" Weast, MA, LPC, NCC, CT
Duke University Cancer Center Patient Support Program

"I'm ecstatic that Joni and Neysa have written this book on how to relate to and live with someone going through a tragic brain cancer diagnosis. Brain tumors can alter emotions, and change any person. Readers will learn how to deal with the emotional side of the crisis. I highly recommend this book to anyone who is dealing with or caring for a person with brain cancer. It is one of the best books I have ever read on this topic."

Katherine Brown, stage IV brain cancer survivor

"I had cancer four times in just four years. This is yet another great 'how to manual' on cancer by Joni Aldrich."

Miracle Mike, terminal cancer survivor, life coach, radio host and motivational speaker

Authors' Page

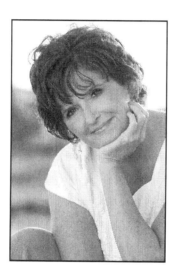

Joni Aldrich, author and speaker. This is the fourth book that Joni has written on how to survive cancer, caregiving, end-of-life issues, and grief. This journey began after she lost her husband, Gordon, to cancer that had metastasized to his brain. She believes that there is an unmet need for practical information to help cancer patients and their families, so she continues to research and write books about the daily rigors of living when cancer invades your world.

Joni believes that she has been prepared throughout her lifetime to write books and reach out to people affected by cancer. Turning her own devastation at the loss of Gordon into hope for others is no easy task, but she believes that she is destined to follow this path.

Neysa Peterson, RN, MS in counseling. Neysa has a wealth of both educational and practical experience with patients suffering from Alzheimer's and dementia. *Patients with brain cancer have very similar brain-altering effects as these patients.*

Through nine years of experience caring for her husband, Jim, Neysa discovered that people with a severe brain illness remain capable of relationships. She learned not to expect Jim to return to her world. Instead, she focused all of her energies on trying to *work within the boundaries of Jim's world,* which is a totally different approach than many families have when a loved one is diagnosed with a mind-altering disease. Jim was still there, and Neysa recognized that. Not only was Neysa able to keep Jim at home until the disease took him, but she also benefited from the daily treasures of love and bonding that many don't know how to facilitate due to the stigma of brain illness. She learned to allow Jim to be a part of the process, instead of making decisions for him. Instead of "you should," she perfected "why don't you?" or "let's try." Neysa's extensive knowledge helped to bring the message of hope included in this book to families dealing with the difficult reality of brain cancer.

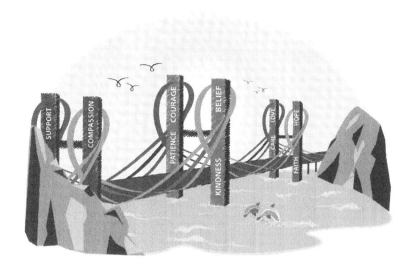

"Bridges" by E. Radomsky

If I could build a bridge to you,

I'd make it straight; I'd make it true,

With lighted lanes and broad expanse,

Without a curve to stumble through.

And when I'm done, across I'd chance,

Like winged dove in spring's romance.

I'd fly like wind and comets bright,

To reach your shores and dance the dance.

I'd never stop, though day or night,

'Til I was home 'neath starbursts bright.

And once alit upon your shore,

I'd burn the bridge and ne'er take flight.

Special thanks to Neysa—
teacher, mentor, and forever friend.

Dedication

THIS BOOK IS dedicated to those who have lived through the experience of having a loved one with brain cancer or are going through it now. I have heard your voice. May our combined efforts connect the realities of brain cancer patients and their families and friends, so that their journey through this difficult disease will be less traumatic for the caregivers and care receivers.

Special thanks to:

Katherine Brown (brain cancer survivor and mother)
Sharon McLaughlin (friend)
Diana DeRosa (mother)
Holly Carson (husband)
Karen Swim (husband)
Cynthia McKay (brother)
Marilyn Randall (husband)
Jeanne Talbot (mother)

Dr. Lee Tessler, MD
Dr. Ravish Patwardhan, MD
Jean Hartford-Todd, CCLS, from the Preston Robert Tisch Brain Tumor Center at Duke University Medical Center

Author's note: It's a privilege—with the aid of Neysa Peterson—to offer this book that can smooth the rough edges for you and your loved one with brain cancer. If I'd had access to this book when my husband Gordon was diagnosed, our journey would not have been fraught with so much pain. This book doesn't have all of the answers, but it does give you tools to build a compassionate bridge between you and your loved one during treatment, and even if facing death becomes a reality. Be strong, and continue to ask God for guidance, peace, and comfort.

Table of Contents

Introduction

I FOUND THIS CYBER SOS posted on CarePages on the Internet, which expresses the desperate need that led to this book:

"Are there any CarePage members out there doing caregiving for cancer victims with right frontal lobe tumors? Besides the obvious 'cancer' issues, there is a lot of coping due to personality changes. I married my soul mate thirty-two years ago, but for the past almost four years I have been taking care of a very different person. We fight the cancer, and we fight with each other. I have problems being the longsuffering wife when I am also grieving the loss of the man I married. Anyone else dealing with like issues? How are you doing it?"

One of the most shocking facts that I uncovered in my research for *The Saving of Gordon: Lifelines to W-I-N Against Cancer* was the high percentage of divorces among brain cancer patients and their spouses. My first reaction—having been the wife of a brain cancer patient—was horror. My second reaction was empathy. Yes, it's shocking even to me. The final weeks of Gordon's life were fraught with painful memories. No, I would never have left him—in fact, I had just loved and nurtured him through two years of hell. The honest truth is that there was a huge amount of emotional damage done to our marriage from the moment that Gordon was diagnosed with brain cancer—for both Gordon and me.

What I really wanted during those dark days was practical information that would help me deal with our greatly altered state of being. A change of strategy was absolutely necessary. Gordon was no longer the man I had known for twenty-two years. Well, he was, but he wasn't. I was weak and vulnerable. Yet no one—not the cancer center, hospital, oncologist, hospice, chaplain, or minister—could give me the guidance that I needed so that Gordon and I could live out those final weeks with the dignity that we had treasured throughout our marriage. Hospice had plenty of information on death and dying, but none on how to deal with the angry, confused, and frustrated Gordon my husband had so quickly become.

No one gave me a crash course in changing from a task-driven caregiver to a brain cancer patient caregiver. I didn't shift gears fast enough. For example, I wanted to be with Gordon every moment that he was awake. But his brain wasn't on my schedule. Consequently, I became more tired and irritable, and I took things Gordon said personally as a direct hit to my emotions. The pain made me more on edge. It was a vicious cycle. I simply didn't know how to get out of it, nor did I have time to focus on what I was doing wrong and how I could handle it better.

The brain is complex, and the heart is fragile. And—when you stop to think about it—*my* thinking mechanism wasn't working at peak performance either. But there were two people involved, and Gordon wasn't the one who could implement the changes. If I had known what I know now, I could have changed to adapt to the different Gordon. Shockingly, I would go through those last horrific weeks before Gordon's death again if I could do so after receiving my coauthor Neysa Peterson's mentoring. That is an astonishing admission.

Upon hearing that your husband, wife, mother, father, sister, brother, child, or friend has brain cancer, no one should go into the days that follow without the tools needed to continue to love and be loved, so that the burden won't be crushing and the "what ifs" will be fewer. What we are going to provide in this book is a gentler approach for loved ones to use while caring for someone with brain cancer.

Author's Note:

Interspersed between chapters are several "Wall of Inspiration" tributes to special people who have had their lives changed by a brain cancer diagnosis and who continue to defy the odds.

The quotes about personal experiences of family members or friends of brain cancer patients were taken from voluntary surveys. These remembrances will help you to realize that your own journey—although different—will be similar in many ways to what others have gone through. I was shocked by the similarities to my experience with Gordon. You are not alone.

We have used these experiences to give you insights so you can understand what is behind the actions of a brain cancer patient and adjust your reaction to deal with the issue more effectively.

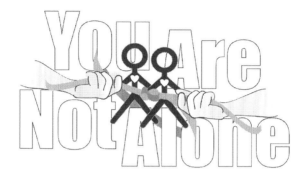

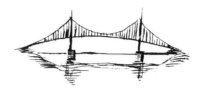

CHAPTER ONE

Bigger Than the Cancer Itself

I N APRIL OF 2006, I stood where you're standing now. My husband Gordon and I had battled tirelessly against the multiple myeloma that raged through his body. We had sparred and parried against every twist and turn of his cancer. Then things started to change in his behavior.

When someone you love begins to show these signs, the first thing we try to do is push it away. It's our imagination. Maybe he or she didn't say what we just thought they said. Or perhaps it's chemo brain. Finally, reality stares you in the face, and action is required. The diagnosis comes that shakes both you and your loved one to the core. Brain cancer—unless it's discovered in the early stages—is more than a cancer diagnosis. How you adapt to the changes will either make it easier in the days ahead or harder.

Which one of us has the brain issue?

While under the influence of brain disease, the patient may as a defense mechanism adopt an attitude that you're the one with the problem. With so much stress and emotion, sometimes you actually find yourself believing it.

Gordon had an innate ability to sound normal, and he certainly looked normal. During the first phases of the disease, you could talk to him for hours and he sounded like the same Gordon. Then an indicator would surface out of nowhere. It had me shaking my head, thinking, "Did I just hear (or see) that, or was it my imagination?"

John Medina, a molecular biologist, published this in the *Harvard Business Review*: "There is no such thing as a perfect memory, because the brain's prime purpose is survival." Part of that survival mechanism early on will have the patient looking at you like you're crazy. The brain is a very complex mechanism that we may never fully comprehend.

"The brain will try to defend itself from threats. Our brains are so complex that it is rare for us to be able to see any situation in exactly the same way as someone else."

David Rock and Jeffrey Schwartz

Often, people with brain tumors are conscious of changes in the way they feel, think, remember, and act. These changes may be so subtle that patients themselves are more aware of them than those closest to them. Sometimes it is the caregiver who first notices the differences. In others, caregivers like my friend Bobbie shake their head years later, and declare that there was never any indication of a brain illness until the patient (her husband) displayed stroke-like symptoms.

Changes may become more noticeable after brain surgery and/or treatment. I've heard, "I took one person into surgery and came out with another." It's not just surgery and tumors that cause issues—radiation, chemo brain, steroids, and antiseizure medications can all put patients at greater risk for cognitive problems.

"The steroids that my husband was on to control the swelling in his brain caused some personality changes. Prior to being diagnosed, my husband was a very patient and loving man. But due to the steroids as well as the frustration from his condition, he became a bit more moody and temperamental. He also experienced a lot of depression."

An important aspect of caregiving for any patient may be keeping a daily journal of behavioral changes, even after the brain cancer diagnosis. It's not about tattling or telling on the patient; it's about their health. However, if you're busy kicking yourself—as I did—for not calling attention to the changes sooner—just stop. We are all simply humans walking a path together with many pitfalls. Here's a remembrance from one of our contributors to the book:

"A year ago tomorrow, we celebrated {our granddaughter} Ava's first birthday. You were hurting badly, and I tried to pretend you were okay. Every second of that day is etched in my mind. I want to mention the night before—our last night together. We were normal—or normal for us. We went to buy Ava's presents. I was gone a lot that month on business, and I didn't notice you were getting sicker by the day. But that night we had a great time shopping. You wanted to get everything in the store. Did you know in your heart that something was up?

"The ride over to Jamie's that day was pretty surreal when I remember it. You drove like a turtle, got lost on the way over to Jamie's, had terrible dry mouth, and your lip was drooping badly. You said weird things like we needed to live close to medical facilities. Do you remember when I said, 'What are we, eighty?' Do you remember when I said, 'It's not like you have a brain tumor'?

"You kept saying you were fine. I blamed your symptoms on the drugs or maybe a toothache—talk about someone in denial. You could barely make it up the stairs to Jamie's living room. But you said you were okay. You slept on the chair, your favorite chair, in front of everyone. But you said you were okay. I kept asking people if they thought you were okay. I knew; the whole day I knew. We would be going to the emergency room, but I just didn't want to go yet, not again. You said you were okay when you drove home; how on earth did I let you drive home? I was really frightened. When we got home, you said you were okay, especially after you self-medicated yourself. You even looked okay. By then I had looked up your symptoms on the Web and became very concerned. I called the ER, and they told me to bring you in. You didn't want to go, but at the same time you knew it was serious. Do you remember filling up my gas tank and saying that this would be the last time? Did you know then?

"We got to the ER; they took us in very quickly. They sent you for a CAT scan, and we received the results right away. I will never forget what

> *the doctor looked like, the expression on his face, or his body language when he told us the news: 'It appears that you have two tumors on your brain, and it looks like it's cancer.' In that one moment—that one sentence, that one expression—our lives changed forever."*

≈

Excerpts from *The Losing of Gordon: A Beacon Through the Storm Called "Grief"*

The weekend before Gordon collapsed, he was driving our motor home seventy-five miles an hour down a busy interstate when I just happened to look up and saw that we were headed straight off the side of the road into the trees. The following Wednesday, we were at the cancer treatment center. Gordon was just walking down the hall, and then suddenly he was falling towards the floor. No, he didn't trip, nor did he pass out. His legs just quit working.

The next morning, we met with Gordon's radiological oncologist. By then, that was the least of my worries. I was trying to tell the doctor that something was terribly wrong. But Gordon was still saying that it was simply my overactive imagination. Thank God he had to go to the bathroom. The minute he left the room, I fell apart and told the doctor that Gordon needed help. He ordered a scan of Gordon's brain. They immediately admitted him into the hospital.

≈

Time to react.

Hours. Not days, weeks, or months. Let's put that span of time in perspective. I had known Gordon for twenty-two years. We were lovers, confidantes, best friends, a strong team, happy campers, and so much more. We completed each other's sentences. While dementia and Alzheimer's patients may have years, a brain cancer patient's mental changes may happen in hours or weeks. Like a thief in the night, the cancer had secreted away some part of the essence of Gordon right in front of my eyes. It had not changed how he looked, or even how he sounded. There were stretches of time where he sounded the same. There were others where he was confused. And the anger was always there, which punched my insecurities in the stomach. Was he mad at me for bringing him home from the hospital with hospice? Or was he just plain mad that now—after the horrific treatments he had endured in an effort to save his life—he was going to lose his fight? We told him he was going to die. As every hour and every day passed, he fought his fate in different ways.

And me—I was devastated. Lower than dirt for giving up on him. As we watched his breaths-per-minute steadily decrease in his hospital bed, I knew he didn't want to die in the hospital. In a last-ditch effort, I called his main treatment facility in Little Rock, Arkansas, and asked—if there was any way in the world that I could get him there—could they do anything? Sometimes reality slaps you in the face. They told me no, that in fact Gordon had been losing the battle for a long time.

So the last weeks of Gordon's life were spent with someone that I barely knew and didn't know how to approach. It took me two years of counseling to get through the scars. It didn't have to be that way for me. It certainly doesn't have to be that way for you.

≈

From Gordon's Perspective

Zero to hallucination.

My name is Gordon. Strange things have been happening to me. I was walking through the cancer center, and I fell down. Maybe I tripped or something. Joni screamed, and all of the nurses ran to help. The doctor came and let me go home. Next day, I was driving to the hospital and my wife got upset with me. She didn't like my driving. We met with another doctor; I told him there was nothing wrong with me. The doctor made me take some kind of medical test. I'm not sure what happened next because everything went blurry.

Three hours later.

I'm in the hospital with crazy things going through my head. I thought I was at the race. Later on, they came and told me something was wrong.

Joni cried a lot. They're going to do a new kind of radiation on my head. More radiation. But the doctor didn't say too many bad things. Joni is usually so strong. She's making calls; I've seen her. I think she's afraid of something. I keep asking for my BlackBerry. I have to get to work. It must be broken. Joni won't bring it to me.

One week later.

I woke up and was happy to be at home. How did I get here? There are all of these people here. They have another bed for me right in the living room. My wife asked what I wanted to eat. I told her a muffaletta. What-ever that is, it tasted pretty good.

Hospice is at our house. Why are they here? I keep asking my wife, and she just cries and cries. I forget why. There are some cats here at the house. I don't know their names. My sisters are here, too. Everyone is so sad. Why are they sad? I'm home.

One week later.

These men came from the church. They asked me if I wanted to pray. I didn't know what to say, but praying seems like a good idea. I can't walk. Everyone says that I haven't been in an accident. They said it's the cancer, but I could walk before. Today my wife asked me where I want to be bur-ied. I've always liked it in Hilton Head. When she said that, I told her okay. While I was eating my sandwich, I thought why not be buried with Uncle Herb? She said okay. Sometimes the pain gets so bad. They're giving me stuff, but it doesn't help.

Another week later.

I feel so angry. Why has Joni given up on me? I still want to fight, but how can I in the wheelchair? I am so helpless. The weather is nice, so they took me out to the front porch. They let me smoke a cigar and gave me a glass of wine. Joni won't let me have too much. I asked her, "What differ-ence does it make? I'm dying anyway." She looked like I had hit her. My sisters are here. That's nice. When I want to eat, I eat these odd ice cream bites. They must be making them, because I eat a lot.

Another week later.

More visitors came. I had a good talk with Chester about cancer and what he can do if he ever gets it. Joni's mom came to stay. I should know her name. I don't sleep at night. Joni's so tired, so she and my sister stay with me off and on. I just want to talk. I tried to talk to Joni about her future. She really cried. I wanted to go in the car. They took me in a bucket truck, and I liked that. I could only go for a little while.

The final week.

I sleep a lot. I don't eat, not even those ice cream things. I asked my sister about taking that tube out where I pee. She said she'd talk to my wife. I feel pain. They give me things. I sleep all of the time now.

Author's note: The events of the day that Gordon was diagnosed with metastatic brain cancer still shake my faith in what I see and hear from other seemingly normal human beings. In retrospect, it was almost as though—once the proverbial cat was out of the bag—Gordon's brain forcefully released the huge flood of negative activity it had been holding behind a stony facade. How else would you explain his tightly held control at eight o'clock in the morning compared to back-to-back vivid hallucinations a few hours later on the very same day? No strong medications had been administered that could explain away the impact of Gordon's full meltdown. The brain is indeed a powerful organ of mental domination.

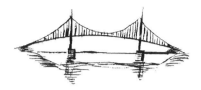

CHAPTER TWO

Faced with an Environment of Change

W ALKING DOWN THE beach today I found a dark purple jellyfish. Technically, it looked more like a big purple blob, but it wasn't a man-of-war and wasn't like anything I've ever seen in my many years of exploring different beaches in our world. Yet there it was, staining the beach purple. I felt somewhat like the M&M in the TV commercial that says, "It does exist!" Simply put, just because I had never seen one before didn't mean it didn't exist. In this book, we're going to enter the land of purple jellyfishes.

As humans, we tend to look at things in black and white. We call it face value. We've learned to form expectations. We work within social norms. When someone you love has brain cancer, things are no longer in black and white—or maybe even in gray. If you can turn your focus away from the black and white, there are other colors to focus on. It certainly doesn't mean that the world is colorless. You just have to find the colors, and they may not be as evident as black and white.

In a big way, I think that what made Neysa so effective with her husband Jim was her ability to step away from the world of normal. For a person *without* a brain illness, that takes real talent. Take for example the times that Neysa found Jim talking to himself in the mirror. He thought there was another person in there. He wasn't frightened as some brain illness patients are—some families have to cover the mirrors in their home.

Jim had found a new friend—he could even reason through the way that the other man got out of the mirror (the back way through the closet). Jim's actions didn't surprise Neysa; she merely accepted it as part of his world.

There's one more thing you need to know about purple jellyfish—they can sting. Being prepared for this fact will make life a little easier. As long as your safety and the safety of others isn't a factor, finding ways to guard your heart against stinging words and behavior may be sufficient to prevent the pain from being too severe.

I want you to picture a cop saying, "Step away from yourself." As you go through changes and unexpected experiences with your loved one, think of yourself stepping out of the "suit" of your old self. Allow yourself to be free of social strictures that may very well have ceased to exist in the world of the person you feel that you no longer know. Freeing yourself of the bonds of the past will allow you to expose yourself more freely to the world that your loved one enters—the land of purple jellyfishes, where we must learn to expect (and in many ways accept) the unexpected.

"Hope for the best, but prepare for the worst."

English Proverb

Now that you are faced with a brain cancer diagnosis, no one can predict what you or your loved one will experience. There's also no way of knowing how long and how extreme the changes you're facing will be. They may be a small wave that you will barely feel, or a tidal wave. Only God knows for sure.

Just to give you an example of the difference in extremes, I have been faced with two different metastatic brain cancer diagnoses in my lifetime: one was Gordon, and the second was recently when my eighty-three-year-old mother was diagnosed. Gordon had multiple tumors throughout his brain. We were blessed that my mother only had one small lesion in her left parietal lobe. Gordon had many different changes in personality and behavior—loss of social inhibition, irritability and anger, memory changes, and so forth. My mother suffered some memory changes (which may have been more related to age than cancer) and some numbness in her hands.

"Many brain tumor patients face changes in memory, thinking, or emotions since the diagnosis of a tumor or its treatment. In fact, studies have documented cognitive impairments in as many as sixty to ninety percent of patients with brain tumors. Patients may experience any combination of changes, and even patients with similar tumors may have quite different experiences."

From the National Brain Tumor Society

Changes in the patient may require that you change, too. And there may not be very much time to adapt. Anticipating the change and understanding why it has become part of your life has the potential to make your journey through your new reality less painful for you, your family, and your loved one with cancer.

> *"Being five steps behind was the biggest frustration when I was trying to be a good caregiver. Each time I adjusted to her current condition, it would change again for the worse."*

There's only one thing you can do—change with the change. And I'd be willing to bet that this caregiver only *felt* five steps behind.

Principles of adaptation:

- ✓ Remind yourself often that you are only human, and therefore imperfect.
- ✓ Create a soothing and comfortable environment for your loved one and for you.
- ✓ Communicating effectively includes listening, interpreting, understanding the underlying emotions, identifying the need, and reassuring the patient through validation of their feelings.
- ✓ Every single day your patient may be different than he or she was the day before. There will be days of clarity, and days of not so

much clarity. Expect the unexpected; appreciate the good days, and patiently work through the bad days.

✓ Meet your loved one in their world. Impossible? Not as impossible as it may be for them to return to yours. Identify where he or she is today, and try to find joy with them there.

✓ Reasoning usually does not work. This may often lead to frustration for both of you because he or she may be unable to follow lengthy explanations.

✓ Never chastise or put down the patient. They are not children, regardless of their brain issues.

✓ Trial and error will require all of your patience and people skills.

✓ No matter what, you can still enrich your loved one's life by creating moments of success and joy, sidestepping moments of failure, and praising their efforts with gusto. After all, aren't these the basic needs that we all require?

✓ Every individual has his or her own unique history, behavior, and personality, a fact that should be held in the utmost respect.

✓ Keep loving the patient *for* their differences—not *in spite* of them.

No right or wrong methodology.

All of my life I've hated to be wrong or make a mistake. It's one of the worst sinking feelings. Now imagine for a moment what it must feel like for the person sitting next to you who doesn't know or understand what they did wrong, or what they could have done differently. They didn't mean to do it. You can't treat them like a child, which I'm sure sometimes we do—even though we don't mean it. When you're impatient or frustrated with your loved one, imagine how they must feel. They might be confused, hurt, or simply closed down.

Now throw into the mix the fact that you—the caregiver or family member—are exhausted and at wits end yourself as to how you can relate and ease your loved one's needs. It's an awful fact that when you need patience the most, your emotional stability will be stretched to the limit. So how do you turn this into a win-win situation?

First and foremost, realize that the patient may not be responsible for their behavior. *Period.* And good or bad, right or wrong, your influence in the *normal* manner (to you) is not going to have a big impact on behaviors and emotions that the care receiver cannot change. Understanding this now, you can start to change your behavior to walk over the bridge to a more peaceful existence. Rest and prayer will prepare you mentally. Centering will help emotionally. For now, plan to change the focus away from your own wants in order to meet your loved one's needs.

The patient may not be able to express the need, but when they hear it from you, they may recognize it as their own. Give these easy questions a try and really listen:

- ✓ What's happening *for* you?
- ✓ What would you like?
- ✓ What would feel good to you now?
- ✓ I hear what you're saying; how can I help?
- ✓ What do you need?
- ✓ What do you think of...?

≈

Keep your heart with all diligence; for out of it are the issues of life.

Proverbs 4:23

The old saying "sticks and stones may break my bones, but words will never hurt me" is not necessarily true. As we all know, words can hurt, especially when our heart is open and exposed. If you don't guard your heart, who will?

Guard your heart. Guarding (not hardening) your heart from potential emotional direct hits inadvertently launched by your loved one will make a tremendous difference. Remember that he or she is probably not acting this way on purpose. Try not to respond with anger or take it personally. Frequently you have to take a step back. Maintain a healthy perspective, and grow through it to maintain sanity and patience. Whatever you do—don't beat yourself up. If you feel you've made a mistake, learn from it and move on. Sometimes a totally new approach is in order. Forget a right answer or wrong answer mentality. I think of it like walking on shells barefooted at the beach—you must step down gingerly before applying more pressure, or you might get cut by a broken shell.

The best method to guard your heart is by hugging yourself. Isn't it amazing that we don't take the time to hug ourselves more often? When words and deeds get hurtful, take your left hand to your right shoulder, then your right hand to your left shoulder. Does this not cover your exposed heart? The signal will mean *stop, think, and regroup*. Perhaps you can even approach it with a smile.

Guard your loved one's heart. By guarding your heart, your loved one will benefit, too. He didn't want to hurt me, but I know that Gordon could often read the hurt in my eyes. He was still the Gordon I had loved for twenty-two years, yet he had lost his personal connection to me with words and deeds. Imagine living with that and not being able to do anything about it to reconnect with the ones that you love.

What will I tell the children?

> *"My son was five years old at the time of her {his grandmother's} illness, and that was difficult for me to explain to him. I wish I'd had age-appropriate information to help me explain brain cancer to him."*

They are the young and innocent. We see them as vulnerable, and our primary focus is to guard them against bad things that happen. But sometimes in the name of protection, we withhold information in the belief that they won't know what's going on. Kids are smart and great at solving puzzles of all kinds. While we can't treat them as adults, we still need to respect their right to understand when life changes are significant—such as when someone they love has a life-threatening and life-changing disease.

Here are the suggestions we received from contributor Jean Hartford-Todd, CCLS, from the Preston Robert Tisch Brain Tumor Center at Duke University Medical Center:

- Let your children know what's going on. Explain that the brain is in charge of all functions of the body. If the brain is damaged, it causes behavior and personality changes, too.

- Acknowledge the emotions your children may have. Help them express their feelings, especially negative emotions such as anger and frustration.

- Practice explanations with your children, so they can answer questions from others without being blindsided.

- Allow time away from the ill patient. This gives the children and the patient a break.

- Set limits with your children as you always have. They must still speak politely and with respect to all family members.

- Provide extra opportunities for active and expressive play. Children often release stress more easily through physical activities.

- Keep your children's school informed. A school counselor or teacher should alert you of any signs of stress that others are observing.

- Model using humor, which can help families cope with difficult times—as long as it's used in an appropriate and respectful way.

- If you feel that the stress is too much for the child, make an appointment with a counselor.

- Be aware and support your own needs, so that you can help your children cope.

I think that the most important message here is that children know so much more and can handle so much more than we usually give them credit for. Yet it has to be presented in such a way as not to traumatize them. If you try to protect them by not keeping them informed, you may do damage in the long term. Work through concerns with love and patience.

The great thing about the "guard your heart" self-hug is that you can teach your children to use it as well. If a parent has brain cancer, there will be times when the children need to know that signal, too. And they get to give themselves a hug in the process.

Wall of Inspiration — Katherine

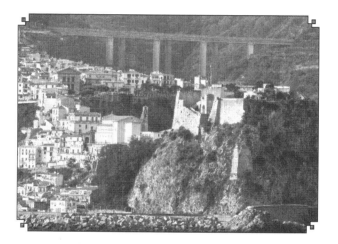

KATHERINE IS A young artist and mother with stage IV brain cancer. One can only imagine the difficulties that this presents daily. But when her back is against the wall, she's tough and knows how to get cooperation from her children, too. See what I mean from her story below:

"When I was going through radiation therapy and chemo at the same time, I started to lose my hair. It really scared my twins (eight years old). Anytime they had a special function at school, they'd beg and plead with me to wear my wig. I had a bald spot on my right frontal lobe area, where they targeted my radiation. As many children do now at an early age, they worried about what their friends would think if they saw me bald with my scar. I would wear my super-cool wig, and that made them happy, but I was completely miserable, as it would impose a ferocious itch. But I wore it anyway for the kids.

"They started misbehaving one afternoon, and I was tired of repeating myself. I shouted out, 'That's it; tomorrow I'll drop you off in front of school without my wig on, and I won't even wear a baseball cap!' They shouted, 'Please don't, Mommy. We promise to be good and listen to you better!' I had found leverage to make them behave.

"Finally, my hair grew back. One day, my daughter said, 'Mommy, your hair has grown back pretty cool.' I thanked her, and then she started to laugh. I asked her what was so funny, and she said, 'Now you can't threaten to take us to school without even your hat on!' I replied, 'Honey, hair is overrated. As quickly as I lost it, I can and might shave my head again when you least expect it!' She just smirked and said, 'That is why I love you so much, Mommy.'"

Author's note:

Katherine's cancer treatment center offers a program called "I Count Too" for children with a parent fighting cancer. It's designed to help them understand what their mother or father will be going through. They tour the cancer facility, and learn about the different types of treatments. Afterwards, all their questions and concerns are addressed.

Katherine's kids then met with a counselor to discuss their feelings. Fears and wishes were placed into their own handmade wish box. The patients are not allowed to be there. Katherine says that she was glad, because her children needed their own "thinking space."

Ask your cancer center if they offer a program like this for your children. The one that Katherine's children attended was structured as a four-week program:

Week 1: Tour of the Cancer Center
Children learn basic information about cancer, treatment and side effects.
Week 2: Fears and Worries
Children engage in activities to help express their worries and concerns.
Week 3: Gifts and Losses
The children explore their feelings and discover unexpected gifts.
Week 4: Hopes and Dreams
The children learn techniques to achieve their dreams.

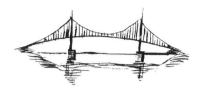

CHAPTER THREE

Preparing for Your Journey

TOPICS RELATED TO the end of life are always difficult to discuss. I was blessed because one of the first things that Gordon did after he was diagnosed was to put his affairs in order. Had I known that he was going to go to the lawyer to do his will, I would have fussed. But it was the right thing to do. That took a lot of courage. He loved me that much.

It is critically important that the following documents and discussions are completed and in the possession of the immediate family:

- Will

- Estate executor

- Trust funds

- Living will

- Healthcare power of attorney

- Rights of survivorship (on all financial accounts, including checking and saving accounts, retirement accounts, and bonds)

- Burial or cremation wishes

- Preferences for funeral services

- Financial arrangements for funeral services

- Documented security passwords to personal accounts online

Don't let this happen to you:

> *"I did not think to keep copies of an important document. It was the document that my brother signed that designated me his medical advocate. When he was placed in the hospital for his final admission, no one could find that I was privy to the information—they could not find the consent form stating that I was his sister."*

> *"I was concerned about what my legal responsibility was to resuscitate him if he collapsed, knowing he had a DNR. I talked to a police officer to determine that in my state, I did not have to comply with his DNR request if he collapsed in my presence. I was told that even EMTs in my state would not comply with a DNR note if {it was} found on an unconscious person."*

Knowing the enemy is key in a brain cancer battle. Malignant *primary* brain tumors originate in the brain and spinal cord. These tumors don't usually spread outside of the central nervous system. Brain cancer from a primary location is a rare type of cancer, and is much less common than metastatic brain cancer. Although tumors can develop in children and adults, they usually develop in different parts of the brain, and therefore have different symptoms.

Metastatic brain tumors travel from cancer in another part of the body to the brain. Many types of cancer can metastasize to the brain, but melanoma, breast, lung, and kidney cancer are the most common. These malignant cells spread through the blood or lymphatic system. Patients and their families with these types of cancers should be alert for changes that could indicate that the cancer has advanced to the brain.

Brain tumors can directly destroy brain cells, or they can damage cells by 1) causing inflammation; 2) compressing other parts of the brain as a tumor grows; 3) inducing brain swelling; or 4) increasing pressure inside of the skull.

Following original diagnosis and treatment, family members and caregivers should be watchful for signs of a recurrence, such as headaches or cognitive changes. It's always better to be safe than sorry, so contact the patient's neuro-oncology care team as soon as possible to address your concerns.

The most common symptoms of brain cancer are weakness, difficulty walking, seizures, and headaches. Other symptoms are nausea, vomiting, blurry vision, or a change in the person's alertness, mental capacity, memory, speech, or personality. Brain tumors can damage vital neurological pathways. Symptoms depend on the location and size of the tumors.

Brain stem: The brain stem is the part of the brain that connects to the spinal cord. It is the pathway for all nerve function from the spinal column to the highest part of the brain. If the brain stem is affected, symptoms may include double vision, a change in facial muscles, nausea, sleepiness, or weakness on one side of the body.

Cerebellum: The cerebellum is located in the back of the brain above the brain stem. If the cerebellum is affected, symptoms may include issues with balance, posture, and coordination, which may result in problems with eating, talking, walking, and moving the eyes.

Frontal lobe: If the frontal lobe is affected, it can cause unorganized thinking leading to impaired judgment, memory loss, changes in behavior and emotions, reduced mental capacity leading to impaired judgment, possible paralysis, impaired sense of smell, and vision loss.

Occipital lobe: If the occipital lobe is affected, it can cause changes in vision, including the inability to recognize things like shapes, colors, or faces.

Parietal lobe: Comprised of a right and left lobe, they control touch, feel, and most importantly comprehension. If the parietal lobe is affected, symptoms include numbness, tingling, seizures, difficulty figuring out where you are, how to get from one place to another, and difficulty recognizing simple things. If the left parietal lobe is affected, the patient can have impaired speech, inability to write, or difficulty understanding what other people are saying.

Temporal lobe: This part of the brain allows us to distinguish smells and sounds, experience fear, and may impact short-term memory.

It may also be helpful to understand the following viewpoint comparing brain injuries (due to illness and/or medical treatments) to other types of injuries:

"Some people believe that when the brain is injured, it can mend completely—like a broken arm. Unfortunately, brain cells do not regenerate like skin or bone cells. Rehabilitating from a brain injury takes time because damaged cells need to relearn how to do things while the brain uses healthy cells to compensate."

From the Brain Injury Association of Minnesota Web site

Treatment decisions.

In making brain cancer treatment decisions, some of the factors your healthcare team will take into consideration include:

- Number of tumors

- Location of tumor(s)

- Size of tumor(s)

- Type of tumor(s)

- Symptoms of the metastases

- Age

- Overall health

- Active primary cancer

Author's note: This book doesn't discuss all of the considerations regarding treatment decisions after a cancer diagnosis. *The Saving of Gordon: Lifelines to W-I-N Against Cancer* can help you with that. But please explore all of your options.

Since available brain cancer treatments are changing and expanding rapidly, always ask your oncologist about new advances—at that or other treatment facilities—that might be an option for your patient. Also note that brain cancer treatment equipment varies widely by facility.

The information below is from American Society of Clinical Oncology Web site (www.cancer.net):

Hyperfractionization: Radiation therapy that uses smaller doses at more frequent intervals.

Immunotherapy: Designed to boost the body's natural defenses to fight the cancer. It uses materials either made by the body or in a laboratory to bolster, target, or restore immune system function.

Targeted therapy: Treatment that targets faulty genes or proteins that contribute to tumor growth and development.

Anti-angiogenesis therapy: The use of drugs to stop tumors from developing new blood vessels. Without blood vessels feeding the tumor with blood, the tumor cannot grow.

Blood-brain barrier disruption: Temporarily disrupts the brain's natural protective barrier in order to allow chemotherapy to more easily enter the brain from the bloodstream.

Gene therapy: Seeks to replace or repair abnormal genes that are causing or helping tumors grow. Researchers are seeking to learn more about the presence, absence, or mutations of specific genes and how they relate to the risk and growth of brain tumors.

Stem cell research: If researchers can identify the stem cells associated with brain tumors, tumor altering may be used as a method of potential treatment in the future.

≈

Throughout your brain cancer journey, emphasize the need for good communication between the healthcare oncology team, the patient, and their family. Express the need to have complete and accurate information regarding: 1) the true scope of the brain cancer diagnosis, 2) the full list of potential ramifications from the treatment options, and 3) where tumors are and the possible impact.

Many of the regrets of people who have lost loved ones to brain cancer—or of those who've survived—are because they weren't adequately prepared for what to expect both in treatments and in the physical and mental difficulties that might result. Gordon's radiological oncologist assured us that if he took the full brain radiation, he had a good chance to beat the cancer tumors in his brain. Three days after the radiation started, Gordon had a bad seizure that set him on a rapid downhill slide.

Ask to speak with others who have had similar treatments, and *always* get a qualified (not cookie-cutter) second opinion.

Here are some other accounts from the families of brain cancer patients:

"My husband had brain surgery, and the neurosurgeon told us that there was a very slight chance that he could lose his speech during the surgery. Unfortunately, he did lose his speech, and we felt afterwards that the doctor had underestimated the chance of that happening. We met many people in speech therapy with the same problems. I know for sure that my husband would not have had the surgery and would have only had radiation and chemotherapy to treat the tumor instead."

"I think we could have used some straight talk about what we were in store for and how best to help her. Mom was big on fighting with dignity, so she wouldn't give in to things like a walker and especially the wheelchair till absolutely necessary."

"I had to fight for small bits of information, and had I known how difficult the process would be, I would have behaved in a much more aggressive manner in order to ascertain the information I was entitled to as his sole surviving relative. I wish I had understood what limited time my brother had left."

"No one in the medical community directly told us her tumor would be fatal. A few days after her diagnosis, we came across a Web site with survival rates for her type of gliobastoma: 0% at twelve months. Fatal, final, and irreversible means fatal, final, and irreversible."

Brain seizures—what they are, what to do, and what to expect.

Normal brain function requires an orderly discharge of electrical impulses. Such impulses enable the brain to communicate with the spinal cord, nerves, and muscles as well as within itself. Seizures may result when the brain's electrical activity is disrupted. About 60% of all brain tumor patients will experience a seizure at least once during their illness. Once started, a seizure cannot be stopped abruptly—most will end naturally. Ask your oncologist about medications to prevent seizures called antiepileptic drugs (AEDs).

There are two main types of brain seizures: 1) Partial seizures affect only one part of the body, such as an arm or leg. Symptoms include twitching, jerking, tingling, and numbness—similar to convulsions. 2) Generalized seizures typically affect the entire body. A person who has this type of seizure can lose consciousness or simply stop moving and become unaware of what is happening. Others might experience violent muscle twitching or spasms. Most seizures only last several minutes (although it may seem like an hour).

Seizures can occur for many reasons in a person suffering from a brain tumor, including increased intracranial pressure caused by the tumor, changes in medication levels, scar tissue caused by surgery, stress, or sleep deprivation.

If you've never seen someone have a seizure, it can be an alarming experience. Here are some tips for helping someone who may be having a seizure:

- Make sure that the person is breathing. Loosen any clothes around the neck.

- Clear the area of any sharp or dangerous objects that are too close.

- Remain calm and call for help. Stay with the person and try to protect them from injury. Place something soft under their head or rest their head in your hands.

- Don't restrain the person (this may cause injury) or put anything into their mouth.

- Lay the person on their side. This is important if the person is unconscious or if they have anything in their mouth.

- Once the immediate danger has passed, seek medical help as soon as possible. Call an ambulance if the seizure lasts for more than five minutes, if the person has multiple seizures in a row, if the patient is injured, or if the person is unable to breathe.

- After the worst of the seizure is past, the patient may be confused. Explain what happened, and let them know that help is on the way.

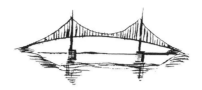

CHAPTER FOUR

Creating a Warm, Comfortable, and Safe Environment

O NE OF THE primary comforts for any patient is a safe place where they can feel at home. Setting the stage with warmth is especially important if your loved one may not recognize their surroundings. Imagine what you would feel like if you were entering that space for the first time. Try to add a little cheeriness to the decor. Creating a warm environment for your patient doesn't mean changing the wallpaper, or pulling the carpet off of the floor. A well-placed photo of a fond memory such as a trip or family gathering will add life and light to any room. Of course, there are other considerations for a brain cancer or critically ill patient.

> *"Mom wanted to stay in bed all the time, but I arranged things so that she had to keep going."*

Whatever the status of your loved one's mental capabilities, *don't give up on the idea that their life can be enriched and meaningful.* That will require some work on your part, but the benefits are rewarding. Simple activities mean a lot. And whatever you do, try to focus on the journey, not the end of the journey.

Safety should always be your first concern. This includes minimizing safety concerns in and around the home, knowing the patient's capabilities for facing the outside world, monitoring driving capabilities, correct administration of medications, and managing nutritional issues.

What you need to be concerned with in and around your home depends on the capabilities of the patient. Gordon couldn't walk, so our concerns were to make sure that he didn't hurt himself in bed or harm himself by trying to get up. If the patient is still mobile, it may be necessary to take precautions like removing matches, firearms, and so forth, or turning off the gas when you're not at home. It may be necessary to confine the patient to a certain part of the house—for example, if you have stairs and are concerned about stability issues. In a sad way, it may seem that you're "childproofing" the house. You may even have to monitor the entry doors.

Regarding medications, it's best to keep them away from the patient. A few dedicated caregivers should have access and control of all medications as prescribed by the doctor. A great pill organizer is essential. Keep doctors and other medical providers aware of any changes in attitude, behavior, and pain level. Maintain an up-to-date record of medications that the patient is taking. If you have to be away from home, have someone else be responsible for administering medications until you return.

For more pleasing surroundings, fragrances (such as perfume or aromatherapy) should be used sparingly and judiciously. The patient's sense of smell may be heightened.

If your loved one can enjoy time outside of the home, be alert for changes in their capabilities. These may be gradual, but they may also happen quickly. Monitor the situation carefully, and ask for others (such as neighbors) to help. It's not about "tattling." We'll discuss more on memory issues and wandering later, but I thought this was a good example of the range of capabilities outside of the home:

> *"Short-term memory problems were common. He had a tendency to forget what he planned to do. Before leaving home, he would ask me to call him on his cell phone within a certain time to make sure he got to his destination. He would call me from the hardware store to ask what he was there to purchase."*

Insights: This actually showed strength on her husband's part because he set up a system in advance to help him remember things. He could then follow the directions that he had asked for. This is a great system for others to accomplish what they need to do—as long as it's safe for the patient and until it becomes an issue.

"When abilities are difficult to recover, patients may learn compensation techniques (i.e., keeping a notebook with reminders to remember appointments, errands, and conversations)."

From the National Brain Tumor Society

As far back as our teenage years, we equate getting our driver's license to independence. While the patient may be able to return to driving at some point, this is one area where the life and safety of not just the patient but of others must be considered. Try to approach it as if it may be a temporary issue. Gordon's decline happened so quickly that this wasn't a battle that we had to face, but under other circumstances I would have had a struggle on my hands. Driving was second nature to him, but the changes in his brain took away his desire to do it.

You may have to be the bad guy, but try not to appear that way to your loved one. One way to do that is to study the laws in your state regarding driving after having a seizure. There are some states that won't allow you to drive for a year. Also, have an occupational driving specialist evaluate the patient. Or make the doctor the heavy.

> *"My husband felt very isolated, which caused depression. Due to his seizures, he was unable to drive, so he stayed home by himself for the most part while I worked. I'm sure it was a very lonely time for him, but unfortunately there wasn't much we could do about it at the time. Occasionally, my father would spend the day with him, but we couldn't do this too often, or he felt like he was being babysat."*

Insights: Having our driver's license makes us feel independent, and that freedom of movement becomes our connection with getting out and experiencing life. If the caregiver is unable to be at home full time with the care receiver, there can be a feeling of isolation. In this example, it would have been nice to arrange for different people to visit, and even take the patient out for a ride or for lunch, if possible. Rotating "visitors" gives a different impression than "babysitting."

The sense of hearing is one of the last to go. Avoid whispering in corners; the patient will know. Don't talk with others in front of the patient as if they're not there, even if they don't appear to be awake. If in doubt, consider how you would want to be treated.

Part of being a caregiver is controlling the stimuli that your care receiver gets from others. Regarding visitors, we are social creatures. The patient's needs and wants regarding company and being out in public should be considered. Educate your family and friends about the disease. Too many people visiting at one time may overwhelm your loved one and upset your routine. Otherwise, encourage visitors because they are very good diversions.

Before friends visit, give them communication tips, such as not asking your loved one too many questions. This can be handled by making others aware of any issues that they may encounter during the visit at the time that they call or come by. You may even want to *let visitors read this book,* so they will understand, too. The key rules that they should be aware of include the following: don't argue with the patient, flow with (not against) the conversation, and ask them to alert the caregiver if the patient becomes concerned or appears to be distressed. Talk with visitors privately after the visit to see if they encountered any concerns that you may need to be aware of.

Out in public people may express how great the patient looks, and we had friends who kept encouraging Gordon to fight. I think that confused him more since I was telling him that his day-to-day fight for life was over. In reality, I failed in my job to prepare those who spoke with Gordon on topics to avoid.

"He was also constantly trying to discuss with people the concept of life after death, and he would get mad if you did not agree with him."

Insights: The patient was passionate, and the topic was definitely applicable to him at the moment. This is a blessing because he believed in life after death. Others should not have argued the point. He was comfortable with the subject. By bringing it up with other people, he was asking them for reassurance, and visitors should have offered him that peace of mind.

On the other hand, if your patient doesn't want to see a visitor, don't force the issue. Follow up with the patient to try to understand, and help them to work through the concerns, especially if it's someone close to the family. It could just be a matter of them not feeling well, or that they don't feel presentable. If there is a legitimate concern, work with them to get it resolved.

"I don't think I had ever considered that there were special people in her life who could not handle her cancer. Some couldn't be with her when she was sick. They just didn't have it in them. It made me more grateful for those who were by our side through it all. I also learned to appreciate those who couldn't be with her by acknowledging in my own mind that they'd had their experiences with her, and nothing would change that. People deal with sickness and death in very different and personal ways."

Insights: This is so true. It's important to realize that people do care, even if they can't visit. Make sure that the patient has thoughtful cards and gifts of love visibly displayed. Also, let the patient know who called or came by while they were asleep.

Surround the patient with things that will bring them comfort (such as photos of family members and pets), whether they're in the hospital, another facility, or at home. Regarding pets, they can be very comforting, although Gordon didn't seem to relate to our cats—whereas they had been one of the centers of our normal life together.

Neysa says that patients with a brain illness do experience boredom. Try to fill the hours with things that your loved one enjoyed before, even if they're not as fast as they used to be. Music can be very soothing. If they were sports-minded, watch the games or listen to them on the radio. While television is a good pastime, you should avoid violent programs— your loved one may have difficulty with making the transition between imagination and reality, so it may frighten them.

> *"Brain cancer cannot rob individuals of their creativity—in whatever form it takes—whereas many other activities and pursuits are limited by brain cancer."*

Insights: Don't focus on what the patient *can't* do. Focus on what they *can* do—especially things that they will enjoy. Gordon enjoyed camping and working. I couldn't exactly build a campfire in the living room of our house or drive the motor home into the living room. But I had a picture of the motor home close by. When he could, we would take him out to the front porch to enjoy the spring weather, have a glass of wine, and smoke a cigar.

Another point of daily focus in our life is food. Forcing the patient to eat is never the answer to assuring a nutritional diet. You'll have to take your cue from them—depending on their situation. Are they in active treatment or palliative care? If they're in active treatment, they'll need to have proper nutrition to fight the cancer. One article said that if you feed yourself, you feed your cancer cells. That didn't sound good to me, but it went on to say that healthy cancer cells are more susceptible to anticancer drugs than undernourished cells. Protein shakes made with ice cream are a great source of strength if the patient refuses to drink other nutritional supplement drinks.

> *"I fed Mom at one point when she could barely eat, and I asked her if she wanted anything else. She said she'd have more for lunch, and we had a mini-conversation about what she would have. But the reality was she wasn't really going to have it. It was life returning, even if for only a moment."*

As in this case, if the patient is in a palliative care situation, your concerns will be different. Do what you can to encourage your loved one to eat, but don't force-feed them. Rather than asking them what they want—which they may not truly know—offer them several choices. Gordon would ask for the "little ice cream things." Eventually, he just stopped eating altogether.

> *"The most difficult aspect was watching a very strong, active man slowly losing his ability to do the things he loved the most. Maintaining my marriage, being a wife even as I stepped into the role of full-time caregiver. I still wanted and needed to be Bo's wife and not see him as a 'patient.'"*

Surround your loved one with love at every opportunity. Try to ignore the many needs swirling around you, and spend as much time as possible with the one that you love—the one who needs your attention. So what if the house is a little cluttered? The primary ingredient in the patient's environment should be your love and attention.

Whispered reassurances to the patient will be good for both of you, even if they seem to be unaware. Nonverbal communications—such as hugging, kissing, or lying down next to them—may give them comfort. A simple touch can offer healing power and is a form of reassurance, a reminder that they are not alone, and a way to offer strength when theirs might be waning. A gentle squeeze of the hand or a comforting touch on the shoulder can work comfort miracles.

Sometimes we don't realize how the little things that we say affect others. Neysa recalls that she and Jim used to work with married couples, and in an effort to heighten their awareness of how their interactions were affecting their spouse, they used red and blue chips. If something the spouse said encouraged them, they received a blue chip. If something the spouse said was perceived as criticism, they received a red chip. At the end of the week, there usually were a lot of red chips! We often say things that are taken as negative by others—especially those with a brain illness. Be aware of the impact of simple words.

> *"He lost all sense of time. He would sit for hours looking at a board game trying to decide on a move to make, not realizing how much time had actually passed. He couldn't make decisions in a speedy way, and sometimes not at all."*

Neysa recalls a morning where she was rushing around trying to get ready to take Jim to a doctor's appointment. She was busily chatting with Jim about everything that they had to do to get there on time. She looked over at Jim and found that he had lain back down on the bed. He then proceeded to tell her that they both knew that wasn't going to happen. In other words, it was a lost cause.

In our world of fast, fast, fast, we expect everyone else to be on our speed. That's not feasible, and it may be hard for the patient to adapt to our time frame. I know it's hard, but it's best to leave some extra time in your schedule so you don't have to rush. Otherwise, your loved one may stage a sit down strike. Try not to push, even though you're in a hurry.

Wall of Inspiration—Seventy-Four-Year-Old Man

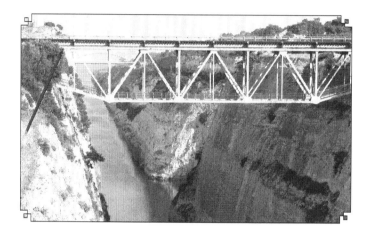

A T SEVENTY-FOUR YEARS old, he is fighting lung cancer, has survived four brain metastases, and has had numerous surgeries and
radio-surgeries. Two and a half years after his initial diagnosis, he
is certainly a patient who can inspire hope.

His neurosurgeon says, "He came to see me in October of 2007 with
speech difficulty. Suspecting a brain tumor, I ordered an MRI that showed
a tumor that had metastasized from lung cancer. I removed the entire
tumor. Post surgery, the patient underwent radiation and chemotherapy.
Fortunately, his speech returned to normal following surgery."

In April 2008, he was diagnosed with a recurrence of his metastatic
brain cancer. The tumor was again completely removed. He remained
without symptoms before or after surgery.

The tumor recurred in the brain again in August 2008. He underwent gamma knife radio-surgery for this recurrence. Although he was still without symptoms, he was diagnosed again with a recurrence in January 2010. He underwent repeat gamma knife radio-surgery.

So how does this patient keep getting knocked down, and still gets right back up? Obviously, he has a tremendous neurosurgeon, who says his patient "takes things as they come—he just has that kind of personality."

The most amazing thing is that this patient remains without headaches or any symptoms two years after his initial diagnosis. Considering the median survival with optimal treatment is ten months with metastatic brain cancer, he can inspire hope in others in this difficult situation.

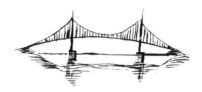

CHAPTER FIVE

Using Effective Listening to Connect

"Listening is the greatest gift one human can give to another. Listening takes time, patience, courage, but is always the right thing to do."

From *Question, Persuade, Refer*, by Paul Quinnett

Never has effective listening been so important. When the patient communicates, it's to fulfill a specific need. He or she wants something, feels discomfort, and/or has feelings or needs clarification about something. Consider the potential cause of unusual behavior. Is your loved one tired, hungry, in pain, frustrated, lonely, or just bored? Could it simply be a side effect of medications? The person who receives the message must then go through the process of interpreting the need with understanding and meaning, even though it may not make sense to them. Effective communication exists between two people when the receiver correctly interprets the sender's message and the emotions behind it. Understanding is half the battle; responding correctly and fulfilling the need is the other half.

There is a big difference between hearing the words that are spoken and really listening for the message. When we listen effectively, we understand what the person is thinking and/or feeling from the other person's perspective. We must be *actively* involved in the communication process and not just listening *passively*.

Open your mind. The old methods of relating to your loved one may not work anymore. No matter what the circumstance, *stay calm*. Losing your patience—no matter how exhausted you are—will build a roadblock instead of a bridge. Think of it this way: if you lose your patience, you lose your patient. They can retreat into their own mind, close it up and throw away the key. That is the last thing you want. Relate in a validating way—one that makes them feel safer.

Try this eight-step method when an unexpected discussion or question surfaces:

STOP (now isn't the time to drop your guard)
LISTEN COMPLETELY (you are looking for clues to the need)
VALIDATION (let the patient know that they have been heard)
CENTER YOURSELF (clear your mind and emotions so you can focus on the need)
DECIDE (this may require asking a question to clarify)
DELIVER THE ANSWER (remember, this may not work on the first try)
TRY A DIFFERENT TACT (if the first answer doesn't satisfy the need)
REASSURE (always a necessary component)

Frustrations for the listener:

- Difficulty communicating by the speaker

- Emotions

- Distractions

- Preoccupation with personal beliefs

- Inability to get clarification

To respond:

- Overcome your emotional reaction.

- Think about your response before you give it.

- Speak as clearly as possible.

- Keep it simple; exclude medical jargon of any kind.

- Avoid giving too much detail at one time.

- Stick to the point.

- Keep body language to a minimum.

- Give your full attention; maintain eye contact.

- Be empathetic, if you can truly empathize.

- Be nonjudgmental on all topics.

- Don't interrupt, or they may lose their thought.

Other considerations of listening:

- Sometimes the person just wants to be heard.

- Look below the surface of the words.

- If clarification doesn't work, use your best guess.

- If the answer doesn't satisfy the patient, regroup and try a different tact.

"We build too many walls and not enough bridges."

Isaac Newton

General tips:

1) Remain flexible, patient, and calm.

2) Don't argue or try to convince.

3) Use memory aids (calendar, pad and paper, write it down, pictures, mementoes).

4) Acknowledge requests, and respond to them.

5) Look for reasons behind each behavior.

6) Consult a physician to identify any issues that may be related to other causes such as medications or the illness itself.

7) Explore various solutions.

8) Don't take the behavior personally.

9) Share your experiences with others.

10) Talk openly to others, but spare the patient any embarrassment.

11) Avoid feeling embarrassed—you are not in a normal situation.

When the subject is pain control, listen even more intently to the concern. Gordon would say, "I'm in so much pain." We would ask him where, but he didn't know, or couldn't say. We would ask if his head hurt (which is probably where his pain was), and he would say no.

I read an article about pain and the brain. It explained that the brain wishes to make sense of the body and its environment. All pain nerves carry signals all the time, but most of the signals don't mean much. The article said we have pain all of the time, but we also have a creative filtering mechanism in our brain so that not all of it gets through to the central processor of sensory information inside the brain. This mechanism is particularly attentive to pain because pain is sometimes the only warning that serious harm is about to occur in the body.

I found this article particularly interesting because in Gordon's final days with the brain cancer, he expressed having more and more pain—so much so that the morphine didn't control it on top of many other painkillers and anti-anxiety drugs. We tried everything. Still, he said that the pain was worse and worse. I have, however, often wondered how much of his pain in those final days was due to actual pain or just his brain telling him that he was in pain. Or perhaps it was the emotional pain—did he want to be out of it and thereby away from reality? When the disease is in the brain, how do we actually know what kind of havoc those mismatched signals are sending? Does it matter if it was real pain or imagined pain? Not when the goal is to make the patient comfortable.

The caregivers and nurses have to be proficient at reading the patient's mood and body language to determine when there is pain and to what degree it's causing them discomfort—especially if the patient is having communication issues. When the patient becomes restless or agitated, they're either uncomfortable or in pain. Body language is 80% of any communication.

> "We (with help from the nurses) had to become adept at reading his mood and body language to determine when he was in pain and to what degree. We could then remind him that pain meds were available, or simply give them to him."

Insights: If the patient is in active treatment, the location of the pain is important. It may indicate an underlying medical condition—such as a bladder or urinary tract infection. Either way, the patient's comfort has to be the number one concern.

When brain cancer is the enemy, caregivers and nurses have to be more creative at determining the cause—and remedy—of the discomfort. Persistent pain is uncomfortable at any level for the patient and their family. With the sheer volume and variety of pain medications available, there isn't a good reason for patients to be in constant pain.

Sometimes cancer patients resist taking pain medications because they fear addiction. This can lead to needless suffering. Simply stated, the difference is that people in pain want medications to feel relief—not to feel drugged. One study showed that out of thousands of cancer patients, only a handful became addicted. Another fear would be concerns about the possibility that the medication may cloud their mind. Healthcare professionals should work with the patient to obtain the needed relief without the loss of alertness.

Pain medications are more effective if the right dosage is determined and then administered at constant intervals rather than on demand. If the right level of medication is elusive, a pain expert may have to be consulted. When Gordon was in active treatment, he had an entire pain management team.

Pain management for brain cancer patients can be tricky. This may include some combination of painkillers and anti-anxiety medications. The goal is both the physical and mental well-being of the patient and as much peace as you can provide. Lean on those who are trained to make the patient comfortable, and be sure that they continue to address the problem until it's solved. Keep them informed of any changes.

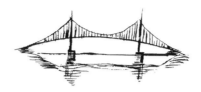

CHAPTER SIX

Patient Communication May Be an Issue

"My husband would get upset with me when I couldn't understand what he was trying to tell me. He hated having to repeat himself, but I would often have to ask him again several times just to understand a simple communication. This caused a great amount of frustration and misplaced anger between the two of us."

YOUR LOVED ONE may have difficulty understanding what you're saying, expressing their own thoughts, or writing. Finding the right words for what they're trying to say is a common problem. It may be a challenge to understand what they need or want. They may also have a short attention span, and may be easily distracted.

Gordon was dying with every breath in the hospital. Once he was settled in the bed at home, he miraculously sat up and said, "I want a muffaletta." Until that moment, I had never heard Gordon use that word. I'd be willing to bet that he didn't know what he was asking for, but I went straight to the only place in town that made that type of sandwich.

While they were in Vermont, Neysa found Jim looking outside at the snow falling on the deserted street. He turned and asked her where the "livers" were. Neysa thought he was talking about meat. She was puzzled.

"Livers?" Jim's sister helped translate: "He's asking where all of the people are that live here."

So now comes the tricky part. When Gordon asked for a muffaletta, there's no way of knowing what he really wanted. He might have meant a ham sandwich or pizza. However, he ate some portion of the muffaletta and was happy with it. It's a good thing he didn't ask for lamb shank when he really wanted a hamburger. The point is this: my take on what he wanted was literal. His probably wasn't. I didn't know. He didn't either. Does it sound like a jigsaw puzzle?

Here are some other examples:

> *"The tumors were in a part of his brain associated with speech, so for a while he reverted to his native language of French, and later spoke a mixture of French, English, and 'word salad.'"*

> *"His loss of speech was one of the most difficult aspects of his illness, since he was unable to communicate his feelings, needs, etc., and this caused him a great amount of frustration and isolation."*

Practice these phrases and use them often to reassure and sooth the care receiver:

- "I love you unconditionally."

- "We're here to help you."

- "We're listening." (This is a phrase that is often underrated and underused.)

≈

The patient may tend to repeat questions that you just answered. Gordon would ask, "Why is hospice here?" I would cry, hold his hand, and patiently explain why they were there. Fifteen minutes later he would ask again, "Why is hospice here?"

Here are some other examples:

> "*Bo would ask what happened to his legs {he was paralyzed}, and I would have to tell him about the cancer all over again. Sometimes he'd look puzzled and ask me again several moments later.*"

> "*My husband was in a hospital, and all he wanted to do was go home. He didn't remember where home was or what it looked like or how to get there, but he knew he wasn't in familiar surroundings, and he knew to ask to go home, so he did this over and over and over.*"

Insights: Keep your answers as simple as possible. A common concern with brain cancer patients is slower thinking speed. Giving them brief answers may suffice, and they will have less to process. Be direct. If they repeat the question again, then you may not have satisfied the need behind the inquiry. There's also another possibility—repeating the same question might simply indicate that the patient doesn't remember asking before, or can't remember the answer that was given.

Try a simple answer first. What I could have tried with Gordon was this response: "Hospice is here to help me take care of you." He might still have asked again, but at least I wouldn't have repeated a long and painful dialogue.

Never argue. You may be picking a fight that you can't win. Worse still, you may be hurting each other unnecessarily. Those disagreements can come back as bad memories. Be clear within yourself about the point you want to get across and find a more effective approach. Choose your battles wisely. Allow the person to control as much as possible, because the number of things they can control may be decreasing moment by moment. Focus on supplying the need, but not embellishing.

Ways to deliver (or redeliver) bad news:

- ✓ Set the stage. If you can, find a place where your loved one is comfortable.

- ✓ Have backup available, if possible. In Gordon's case, I should have used his sisters more effectively. It never hurts to ask, "Who else would you like to be here for this discussion?"

- ✓ Set up a two-way conversation by asking something like, "How are you feeling right now?"

- ✓ Find out how much the patient knows already. Ask, "What have you already been told?" Often, what they know depends on what they want and need to understand for their comfort.

- ✓ Give the information in small chunks, and be sure to stop between each chunk to ask the patient if he or she understands. Ask questions regularly. Long lectures are overwhelming and confusing.

- ✓ Pause to understand how your loved one is feeling. You may be more nervous and anxious than they are. Never miss an opportunity to be caring, but this may not be a time for empathy since you don't know how they feel. Simply ask, "How do you feel about this?"

Never presume. Don't say things like "I know how you feel" or "I'm sure you would feel better if you did this." Presuming you know how someone feels is a sure way to close the door on further communication. But it's always okay to say, "Help me understand," or "What can I do to help you?"

Wall of Inspiration—Sixty-One-Year-Old Woman

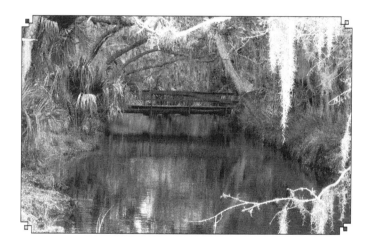

I N 2008, SHE was diagnosed with early stage breast cancer at the age of sixty-one, and she had a lumpectomy and radiation. She was on the road to recovery until October 2009, when she began having difficulty reading, writing, using numbers, as well as mild speech problems. Her main complaint was that she couldn't read to her grandchildren anymore. An MRI showed a tumor in the area of the brain responsible for speech and a number of higher cognitive functions. Her diagnosis was glioblastoma multiforme, the most aggressive of all primary brain cancers.

The neurosurgeon determined that the entire tumor would need to be removed. One short week after the surgery, the surgeon's wife was surprised to find her at the beauty parlor bragging about the fact that she'd had brain surgery just the week before. All of her symptoms thankfully disappeared. Her doctor notes that it's important to get up and around and back into life, as long as the patient doesn't overdo it. Post recovery, she underwent radiation therapy.

Then in 2010 another blow came. She was diagnosed with stage I uterine cancer, had a hysterectomy, and is currently undergoing chemotherapy. She remains without neurological symptoms.

A study in courage and perseverance, after being diagnosed with three cancers in a little over a year, this patient continues to fight them all. Where does she get her spirit and mental strength? "She has a strong family support system."

The neurosurgeon admits that—with cancer on so many fronts—this woman may not live her normal lifespan. But the treatments that they've focused on are for quality of life, not necessarily longevity. There has to be a balance between the two.

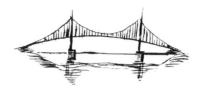

CHAPTER SEVEN

The Line Between Lack of Inhibition and Simple Innocence

W HAT IS INHIBITION, and how has it become important to you? Prior to being enlightened, my idea of uninhibited was when someone threw off their clothes and ran down the street naked— not as an exhibition, but in the sense that a child would do it. Social inhibition is a limitation or curbing of an action, statement, or behavior by a person. Basically, it is our screening mechanism that keeps us from hurting each other's feelings.

We are taught social inhibition almost before we say our first words— right after "Mom" and "Dad," it's say "please" and "thank you." Brain cancer patients may lose the social niceties we're used to, which may make them abrupt, rude, and even sometimes inappropriate.

Inhibitions allow us to fit into social norms, thus reducing or preventing antisocial impulses from being acted on. The perception of what is and isn't socially acceptable may vary in each of us. For example, would it bother you to eat at the table with someone who grabs something off of other people's plates—not rarely, but frequently?

The symptoms may be purely innocent. Neysa's husband Jim was a very appropriate guy. He worked with people as a professor and counselor for many years. In his illness, he would more innocently express his thoughts, such as calling children and waitresses "cutie." Asking him to change the behavior wouldn't have helped; in his mind, he hadn't done anything wrong. In this age of sexual awareness, Neysa was concerned that someone might be offended. They never were. He wasn't invading their space, and when they saw Jim they had a sense that it was indeed innocent. If she felt the person was uncomfortable, she would either discreetly take them aside to explain, or she had these preprinted cards she could hand to them.

> **Please pardon my companion who has dementia.**
> **Any unusual behavior is due to the disease.**
> **I appreciate your patience and understanding.**

> *"He actually became more affectionate as he became more ill. He wanted someone lying next to him in bed as much as possible. One time I came into his room at the care center to find a caretaker in bed with him. He wanted her to lie beside him to watch a movie, and he was there with his arm around her as if it were me. It was inappropriate for her to be in bed with him, and she nearly lost her job over it, but this is something he would never have done if not for the illness."*

Insights: Although seemingly innocent, I can only imagine how unsettling this was! First, you must find out what the need is and determine how it can be met. Was it because the patient didn't want to be alone? Once you discover the need, look for something that will fill the void when you can't be there—other than a healthcare provider. It might be as simple as a body-length pillow to hold or a safety blanket. Offer it by saying, "Here is something to keep you company until I return." If your loved one is in a healthcare facility, you may still be able to have some alone time and privacy. Have the facility put a "do not disturb" note on the door. Otherwise, appreciate innocent needs for what they are—unless they are truly inappropriate.

One night when he wasn't able to sleep, Gordon told me that he was in love with another woman—someone he worked with. For one moment in time, I thought my ever-faithful husband might have been confiding in me about a deep, dark secret. But I knew the object of that love, and I realized immediately that he was talking about the innocent love for another human being. The way he phrased it, though, he had me going for a minute. But trust me, it could be worse. I have a friend who found out that her husband had a brain illness because he was around town picking up prostitutes!

Another night Gordon said, "We need to discuss what's going to happen to you for the rest of your life." He said it with almost a nonchalant attitude. I immediately broke down. He then shocked me by shouting, "Oh, just grow up." This was a man I had spent the last two years trying to save through some of the worst challenges imaginable!

Insights: I understand now that this conversation showed the depth of Gordon's love for me; he was worried about what was going to happen to me after he died. Unfortunately, without inhibitions, it was delivered in a harsh way that hurt my already bruised spirit. Neysa believes that he had probably been walking on eggshells to get the courage to have this conversation. When I broke down, he responded out of frustration. I didn't have my heart guard up, so I cried alone all night. It was a giant shove into the grief process. As I was still somewhat in denial, I wasn't prepared to discuss this with him. Neysa phrased it this way: "You caught the ball before you saw it coming, and it had already made contact." In reality, it was worse than that. I didn't believe he had the emotional or mental foresight to approach that serious topic. When he voiced it in such a nonchalant way, it lacked the sharing comfort we had developed over our many years together. And—worse still—as a natural part of anticipatory grief, I had already been agonizing about my future without Gordon. What he said hit a "guilt wall." If I had been prepared, appropriate responses would have been: "Would it be alright to talk about this tomorrow when I'm not so tired?" or "What would comfort you for me to know?" or "Have you been thinking about that?"

"Before the paralysis, Bo went out into the yard and cut down tree branches like a mad man. When I asked what he was doing, he told me that he was not going to be around, so he needed to trim the trees for me. While it was a typical loving gesture, he knew how much I loved him and believed he would live. In a normal mindset, he would have spared my feelings."

Insights: This is also a sign of love; Bo was doing things in advance. Just as in my case, the receiver wasn't prepared for his abruptness. His comments were no doubt out of frustration. Men like to be in charge of things. There are certain things that they believe are their responsibility to do—like yard work. I saw this in Gordon often as the cancer took away his ability to do things like wash the motor home and change the oil. It's hard to watch someone taking over your responsibilities. A loving, caring response would be, "Thank you for thinking of me." Too often, our emotions get the better of us, and we forget to pull up the heart armor, especially when it's a surprise attack. You might add, "Is there anything else that I should be prepared for?" Or just simply pick up the wheelbarrow and help. Sometimes, physical exertion is good for the soul.

"As I realized that Brian was nearing death, I escalated visits, oftentimes going from Denver to Florida every three days. As his illness progressed, I called him and asked if I could come down in the next few days. He replied that he didn't want me spending my money on flights and hotels. And then he added, 'Besides, there is nothing to do here.' It broke my heart as he was my primary concern during the time of his illness, and I desperately wanted to spend time with him."

Insights: If you feel that you need to go, just go. If you must tell them in advance, just say, "I'm coming down." Follow that with, "I really want to be with you." It sounds like the brother was trying to take care of the sister, which is the case the majority of the time. Loved ones don't want to be a burden. Accepting gifts of love like extensive travel expenses may be hard to accept because the favor can't be repaid. Just go; if they continue to argue, tell them that you're doing this for your own peace of mind.

> *"One event happened in church. In an effort to stress how awed he was at the sacrifices of Jesus, he repeated several times to me that 'Jesus was f**ing awesome!' in the middle of Mass."*

Insights: The message wasn't delivered too well, but it showed great depth of spirituality. Neysa said, "At least he didn't go up to the pulpit and take over the sermon." Unless people are offended, allow your loved one to be spontaneous. If they are offended, then you may have to give out dozens of explanation cards. If the patient persists in being disruptive, perhaps you shouldn't take him or her back to that setting. The bottom line is, try to have a sense of humor, even if it seems inappropriate to you. Yes, I know it was church, but it doesn't appear that he was truly being disrespectful of God—quite the contrary!

> *"He swore more than usual after the cancer diagnosis and radiation treatment. He wanted to talk to elderly people about dying, even if it was at inappropriate times and in inappropriate places."*

Insights: The swearing would indicate frustration and lack of inhibition, but it's a difficult issue to change in this case. If possible, in cases like this you should control the people the patient is around, or hand out explanation cards. You can't change the behavior, so create an appropriate environment.

Death is not always a comfortable subject for people, especially in the wrong setting. On a positive note, he was evidently comfortable talking about death. But, what was the need he was trying to fill? Was it reinforcement or curiosity? Maybe it would help to create a setting with people *of common beliefs*, so that he could discuss it openly until his needs are met. If the expectations surrounding death are negative, counseling may be called for.

> *"My husband exhibited loss of inhibitions later on in his illness. By that time, he was so tired of doctors, etc., that he didn't care who saw him naked. There was one time that I came home from work and found him lying on the floor next to the bed, so I called 911. He was rushed to the hospital (naked). Once he came to in the ER and was more coherent, he decided he wanted to go home immediately, but we had no clothes there for him. Thankfully, my parents rushed back to the house to get his clothes; otherwise, we truly thought he would have left the hospital naked."*

Insights: Remember when I said, "Allow yourself to be free of social strictures that may very well have ceased to exist in the world of the person you might no longer know"? In this case, there's only an issue if the patient is upset about it. While we strive to protect our loved one's dignity, the healthcare community is used to these types of issues. And it didn't seem to bother the patient one bit.

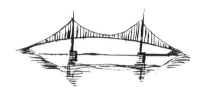

CHAPTER EIGHT

Changes in Personality, Behavior, and Emotions

C HANGES IN THE person you once knew—no matter how extreme—are not reflective of the true person inside, but of the disease process itself. Brain tumors can affect the thinking skills, emotions, and/or personality. Problems with memory, speech, and/or concentration may occur. Your loved one may have serious mental challenges complicated with confusion. Moods may change often. The person you knew may act differently than they acted before and may have difficulty doing more than one task at a time. Check with the doctor to find out about treatments that may help.

Anger from your loved one may come from frustration. It's like turning up the volume on the radio—they want to be heard. You've heard the old saying that the squeaky wheel gets the grease? If you *hear* the need, the patient feels that you'll try to do something about it.

As a caregiver, family member, or friend, you may choose to receive counseling to: 1) learn how to help your loved one deal with the mental changes they are having, or 2) learn to deal with your own reactions to changes in your loved one.

> *"In the months leading up to his initial diagnosis, my husband started to abuse alcohol, becoming embarrassing to be with, belligerent, rough, and mean, the opposite of the man I fell in love with. The last straw came when we were on a trip celebrating our one-year anniversary. My mild-mannered husband drank one evening away and became verbally abusive and physically threatening. I spent the night locked in the bathroom; I was afraid he would hit me. When we returned, a doctor's visit caught the tumor. It was such a relief when the first surgery gave him back to me."*

Insights: This woman is a very brave person, but in some ways she put her safety in jeopardy. If the behavior is aggressive, back away. Give your loved one some space. Then calmly approach him or her. Don't argue. Regardless of how much love you feel for the person, you have to keep yourself safe. Don't assume that you know the reason for the behavior. In this case, the alcohol was the detonator. The tumor had robbed him of any abilities he had to control his behavior. Thank God the tumor was found before someone got hurt! Above all else, protect yourself and others, protect your heart, and find out what's going on.

> *"Brian became withdrawn and only wanted to read, which was unusual for his normally outgoing personality. He became somewhat antisocial as well."*

Insights: It may be that the patient didn't have the energy to be gregarious and outgoing. A withdrawing reaction in people is similar to hibernation for animals—we tend to draw up into ourselves to allow time to deal with the situation. Antisocial behavior can simply be a lack of willingness to think of other people's needs so that you can focus on your own. Be as supportive as possible, but continue to give them opportunities to interact with others in a controlled setting. Don't push the issue. It is, however, important for the caregiver to maintain contact with other people. The question becomes how to take care of the patient's needs and your needs, too. Quality of life applies to both the patient *and* caregiver.

> *"He would get out of bed during the night and begin to dismantle furniture or equipment around his living area. He was destroying things that all of his life he loved and cared for."*

Insights: In a situation like this, you should try to find out why the patient is awake at night. Talk to their doctor about a sleep aid. If a similar situation arises for you, ask your loved one, "Why are you doing that? You made these things, and they're so right—why do you want to take them apart?" It could be anger. If you can connect with the emotion behind the behavior, you'll know how to respond. We usually focus on the emotion first, not the behavior. Talk with your loved one in a compassionate way. Feelings aren't right or wrong— they just are what they are. In the example, the patient might have thought he was being helpful—things are easier to move when they're dismantled.

> *"He would say things like, 'I smoked buildings for a living' (he was a retired fireman), and he was going to smoke because it didn't matter anymore—he was dying anyway."*

Insights: When brain illness is the problem, the patient is less able to gain victory over an addiction. His statement reflects the feeling of helplessness. In a situation like this, you can ask the patient, "Would you like some help to deal with that?" or "Help me to understand what that feels like." Understand that the issue is not about you. Maybe the patient just needs someone to listen. Truthfully, *you don't know what it feels like to know that you're going to die.* To release the pressure, the patient may lash out in anger. Other times they may be able to talk with you reasonably about it. Don't focus on *you* in cases like this—give the patient a safe environment where you won't deny or judge them.

> *Gordon wanted wine for breakfast, which I refused because I was afraid that the medications and alcohol could cause an overdose that could kill him. He asked, "What difference does it make? I'm dying anyway." In his normal state, he would never have hurt me that way.*

Insights: Don't discount the person or the need. I was still looking for things in the reality-based universe. Maybe I pushed Gordon into giving a negative, angry response—one that I wasn't prepared to address. Hearing him talk about dying so bitterly was a direct hit to my emotional core. I lacked the comfort level to realize that the issue wasn't about me. Perhaps if I had taken that moment to open up and address his anger, we might have cried together. It's sad, but I don't remember him crying that much. I was too busy trying to deal with my emotions. Know that the issue is not about you. Tell them that you're listening. It is evidence of unreleased pressure when your loved one blurts out their anger. Other times they may be able to talk with you about it. Take your cue from the patient. Try to take your feelings off the front burner. Be the bigger person, and then count to ten and leave the room for a minute if you have to.

One of our contributing neurosurgeons noted that steroids and antiseizure medications could cause behavioral changes in the patient. If personality changes are extreme, the medications that a patient is taking should be considered. Discuss any concerns you may have with a doctor.

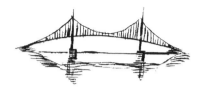

CHAPTER NINE

Memory Changes and the Resulting Confusion

I MAGINE WAKING UP with amnesia and not recognizing anything or anyone around you. It takes years to store our precious memories, but then we can lose the links to them sometimes instantly due to various causes—one is brain illness. Yet, what remains when the links to those memories are gone? There may be more than you think.

> *"Instead of waiting for me after one session got out early, we found him wandering around the neighborhood next to the facility. He was found several times wandering our own neighborhood while I was at work. Luckily, neighbors recognized him and made sure he got home safely."*

Insights: The first time that the patient wanders while looking for something familiar can be a wake-up call. Neysa recommends that caregivers try to ascertain what the patient is seeking or needing. In some cases, it's an indication that a physical or emotional need is not being met. It could be that they're curious, bored, or looking for something. "Wandering for a person can be an indication that they need to be more active than they're being allowed to be." With proper supervision, wandering can be a great way to get exercise and a pleasure for the patient. Go with them or follow at a safe distance. Intervene when they appear to be getting tired. If they're capable, take them to the gym, a mall, or somewhere that they enjoy. It helps them feel active and can be a break from staring their illness in the face. At some point, supervision may not be enough, and wandering can be a problem. One solution is a tracking device—usually a bracelet, but they also have shoes. If the patient is missing, they can use GPS to determine their exact location.

Using routines to counteract memory loss.

Have you ever turned the light out while leaving a room even though there were others still in there? Or even worse, have you done it when the electricity is out? Habits are a part of a different area in the brain that tends to remain intact longer than regular memories. If you can set and keep routines, your loved one doesn't have to stop and think about what to do next. Examples include eating breakfast before getting dressed, sitting in the same recliner in the living room each morning, and taking a bath in the evening.

As a caregiver, you need to know your patient's daily rituals. And you're in a unique position to customize and refine the routine so that it includes meaningful activities. These daily activities may seem insignificant from your perspective, but they add depth to your loved one's day and provide him or her with activity. These may include: 1) personal hygiene; 2) meal-time preparation, serving, eating, and cleanup; and 3) household chores. If the patient can help in these areas, it gives them a sense of purpose and will help you out, too!

If the patient is physically capable, part of this routine should be regular exercise. Exercise may help improve both the brain-related symptoms and quality of life. Studies have shown that physically active people exhibit higher levels of cognitive functioning than inactive people. The theory is that physically active people have a "cognitive reserve" that is used when other areas of the brain are damaged.

Around the house, you may need to remove distractions and limit choices. This may mean narrowing the choices for dinner or the number of clothing options. It also may mean relocating an item in the house that may otherwise cause your loved one to become distracted from the task at hand.

You should reexamine routines frequently—especially if you notice that the patient is agitated, unsettled, or depressed. There may come a time when you can't sustain even basic routines. At this point, flexibility is important. Caregivers should step down expectations according to changes in capabilities.

Stay flexible. You can't schedule every activity and event in advance. When an unexpected or unforeseen change occurs in the routine, just restart your routine the next day.

Other suggestions:

- Keep a calendar of activities visible on the wall. Cross off days as they pass.

- Frame and label pictures of family members, friends, home, and so on.

- Actively include the person in family activities and conversations.

- Limit alcohol use, contact sports, sharp objects, driving, and cooking without supervision.

≈

One day your loved one may ask, "Who are you?"

When we're born, our parents name us based on their favorite names. By no means does that title make us who we are inside and outside. Yet one of the first things that people will tell you after a visit to a nursing home to see their ninety-year-old grandmother is, "She didn't remember my name!" It can be very disturbing when someone we love forgets our name. But have they forgotten who we really are? Maybe, maybe not. According to Neysa, they usually haven't forgotten the essence of who you are.

I was appalled when Gordon couldn't remember my mother's name. She's my mother! But was it that important? He remembered *her*, just not her given name. He still interacted well with her. There was still love. He had just lost the connection to the name "Martha" as who she was.

Neysa's experience with Jim regarding who she was has a different twist. He began to know her as the woman who lived there, and he even thought she was a different person upstairs and downstairs (I guess it was good they didn't have four floors). He asked her once, "Is the woman that lives downstairs there?" She tried to explain that there wasn't anyone downstairs, but that didn't satisfy his curiosity, so she asked him to go see. He went and was satisfied that there was no one there.

> *"Rob's memory only became bad the last few months. He would forget friends' and nurses' names, and he couldn't recognize his father; the last two people he could remember were me and our son, Jack."*

Another spouse said this about her husband with brain cancer: *"He went through one time when he thought that I was his ex-wife and even called me by her name."*

Insights: Have you ever remembered the face of someone, but not the name? It will drive you crazy until you figure it out. They are in your mental picture bank, but you just can't connect a name with a face. That's similar to what the brain cancer patient is experiencing. Your loved one continues to know much about you, even if they have forgotten your name—or call you by their ex's name (admittedly that would be disturbing). You are familiar and have a close history with them. In some cases, they may remember the names of those closest to them, but not the less frequent visitors. If he or she doesn't see a person every day, they may not remember them. However, they can maintain the context in which the person is important in their existence.

Memory capabilities may diminish over time. You can help—ask visitors to refresh the patient's memory by mentioning who they are when they first arrive. They should communicate that information at eye level to deliver the message more effectively. If the patient still doesn't recognize them, request that the visitor resist responding with hurt feelings or saying something like, "You know who I am, don't you?" Instead, reassure the patient that it's okay.

First and foremost, remember that it is a choice that you or others are making if you allow yourself to feel hurt when your loved one forgets your name.

≈

Don't fight the memory.

> *"My mom would have very vivid memories that she would believe were happening right now. She would ask me, 'Don't I look beautiful in this dress that Marge bought me when she was in China?' I knew the dress because I had seen it in pictures as a child. It was gorgeous, and my mom did look gorgeous in it. She was probably in her twenties when that special dress was given to her. At first, I was confused about these comments, but then I realized that I wanted to be part of those memories with her. So I joined her memory and helped make it reality for her. 'Yes, you look gorgeous. Where are you going? Who's going out with you?' I would ask her questions about it, not as her daughter, but as part of that experience."*

Insights: This daughter gets high praise for sharing this special moment with her mother. Obviously, it was poignant for both of them. So what if it wasn't a then-and-now memory? It was still meaningful and beautiful. Not only did the daughter share the memory, she facilitated the fantasy so her mother would be happy. What a great gift.

≈

Loss of "home."

> *"My mother was absolutely convinced that she was not in her house and that my dad was absolutely not her husband. She would say, 'This is not my house. I know this is not my house. Please take me home.' She would call for my dad, 'Dick, where are you? Please come and get me and take me home!' My dad would be standing with her trying to reassure her that she was home and that he was Dick. He was her husband."*

Insights: One effective method for troubling behavior is to act like you agree, thereby connecting with them, and then distracting the patient away from the issue. If the cat that you don't have needs to be put out, go ahead and do it. When you interrupt the behavior, you don't gain an understanding of why it is important. For example, if your loved one constantly heads to the door asking to go home, efforts to try to distract him or her may not work. Try something like, "I know you miss your family." Afterwards, sit down and look through family photo albums. You've acknowledged the concern and enacted a solution, which will possibly sooth the need.

This reminds me of a story Neysa told me about Jim. He decided that "someone" was coming to steal the house—not just things from the house, but the whole house. She tried to reason with him—the first line of defense, although often useless—and explained that it was impossible to steal a whole house. When that didn't work, she tried a different tactic: "Jim, if they come to steal the house, I'll just call the police, and they'll take care of everything." Jim respected the transference of the concern to the authorities, and he was satisfied—the subject never came up again. Neysa had effectively resolved Jim's anxiety.

So what would have happened in the "loss of home" scenario if—instead of fighting the problem—the daughter and husband had worked within the memory? Perhaps they could have said, "We're taking you home very soon." Or they could have reassured her that they were going to get her husband right away. In our daily walk in life, we are used to being so grounded—is that why it's so hard to let go? Use your imagination. If you find a tactic that works, stick with it. Don't continue to try the same approaches that aren't working. You know the old saying: "If at first you don't succeed, try, try again."

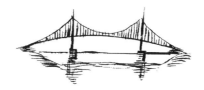

CHAPTER TEN

Questions about Brain-Related Paralysis

S INCE HE COULDN'T walk, Gordon asked if he had been in an accident. Isn't an auto accident or a falling accident what we expect to lead to paralysis? We don't anticipate a brain tumor. It was as though the two years we had fought against his cancer hadn't existed. Since he had spent so much of his life driving vehicles, the loss of mobility probably solidified his worst nightmares from the road. When he asked, we told him no, that it was the cancer. That only seemed to confuse him more. It was probably too much for him to deal with.

> *"My husband would ask why he couldn't move his legs. The cancer had spread to his spine, and he was paralyzed from the waist down. Although he knew that, I would have to recount the story of what happened."*

Insights: Patients are trying to come up with an explanation themselves, so share the truth with them in a simple way. Encourage the thought—for example, you might say, "Honey, it's great that you came up with that possibility, but that wasn't what happened." Hopefully, that will ease their fears. Try attaching the cause to a memory (such as being in the hospital) that they might relate to. Don't make a big deal out of it. Attempt (at least once) to orient him/her to the true reality. If that doesn't work, try saying, "It seems like you've been thinking about that," to distract them, and then divert the issue. Consider that this may also be an opportunity to reassure them, and allow them to talk openly about their concerns. Try one of the following:

- "No, there wasn't a car crash, but I can understand why you might think that."

- "It's okay to feel what you're feeling, and I can see where you came up with that."

- "Are you asking if you're going to get better?"

> *"He was terrified of me bathing him after the paralysis. We had the bathroom completely outfitted with the bars and shower seat, but he was so scared (completely unlike him) that some days I would have to bathe him in bed."*

Insights: It's hard to know from this explanation, but I have to wonder if the patient had an unspoken idea that a fall in the bathtub had caused his paralysis. Darlene, another friend who had metastatic brain cancer, had believed that. While you may never know the cause of the distress, you can try a less terrifying alternative, such as bathing in bed.

Some brain illness patients exhibit an irrational fear of the bathtub, water, or personal exposure. Ask a healthcare provider or hospice nurse what they recommend. There is nothing wrong with bathing the patient in bed. Try to make the environment comfortable—for example, provide warm blankets. Use baby towels, which are softer. If the fear is related to water specifically, try no-rinse soap. The nurses may recommend that you can wash different sections of the patient's body on different days, if bathing distresses them. One bath a week may be sufficient, unless the patient is active. Again, don't take it personally. Caregivers should be patient-oriented, which this wife was when she recognized the issue and changed the strategy. If you're task-oriented rather than patient-oriented, you may push too hard, invade their space, and push your loved one away.

"My husband thought he was invincible and felt nothing he did could or would hurt him. He couldn't walk upright without falling every few steps, but he would just keep trying as if nothing had happened. He never saw the falling as a symptom of a problem. He accepted it as if it were normal for him."

Insights: When faced with this situation, safety is the bigger issue than pride. You must maximize the safety and minimize potential injury to the patient. Ask yourself why does he want to move? Could you bring something to him? (Make sure that all items he regularly needs are close at hand.) Would rehabilitation with an occupational or physical therapist help with the mobility issues? While restraining the patient may not be an option, can you limit them to a specific "safety" zone?

Taking precautions to ensure safety may include the following:

- Remove obstacles, breakables, tripping hazards (such as rugs), and pad the floor with something like that puzzle padding used in children's rooms.

- Keep them away from stairs, even if you have to limit their living area.

- Try to get the patient to wear a helmet, kneepads, wrist pads, and so forth. Can you make an adventure of it?

- If you feel that the patient should be supervised whenever they're up, try to get a hospital bed with alarms, or put a mat alarm next to the bed.

- When the weather is nice, offer movement in a less painful environment, such as a lawn where the grass is soft.

- Make sure that clothing isn't too baggy and that shoes fit well and have nonskid soles.

- Make sure that rooms are well lit, even in the evening.

"*Mom would ask to hold the water glass herself, but she was incapable of doing that. I think when she realized that and that she could not stand is when she gave up.*"

Insights: We learn these things at a young age. When we lose them through illness, it seems so unfair. In a situation where the patient can't hold a glass, you might try straws or a non-spilling sippy cup. Try to keep as much normal in the patient's life as you can, but the loss of the ability to perform simple tasks that they've done all of their life may be depressing. Focus on what you can do to change the things that are changeable, and offer support and love for everything else.

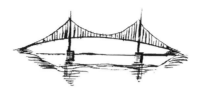

CHAPTER ELEVEN

Coping with Impaired Judgment

W E KNOW THAT our brain controls everything that we do, say, think and feel. When it's not functioning at peak performance, issues related to behavior can result in poor choices by the patient. Caregivers and family members may need to address mental changes quickly as they become apparent.

> *"My husband was seen picking up used cigarette butts out of public ashtrays outside of businesses. He was using matches and fire in unsafe ways."*

Insights: This is both a health and safety issue. A patient like this needs close supervision, especially when around used butts or matches. If they took away his cigarettes, what would be the ramifications of allowing him a supervised cigarette (of course, without giving him possession of the matches)? Safety issues dictate that you have to keep all matches out of his reach—locked away and where he can't burn the house down. There are pieces of this story we can't know, such as: 1) What did he say when he was asked why he was doing it? 2) How did he react to being chastised about it—what was he wanting? 3) Were they allowing him to smoke in a supervised way? 4) Had they tried nicotine patches or other smoking cessation products?

> *"My husband had lost his voice to larynx cancer and his lung to lung cancer, and he still continued to smoke."*

Electronic cigarettes are a good alternative to smoking. They look, feel, and some even taste like a real cigarette, and they require the same mechanical motion of smoking. The unit emits no real smoke—the discharge is an almost odorless and definitely harmless water vapor that looks like smoke. In the front of the device is an operating mode indicator that lights up when you use it and simulates the burn of a cigarette. And the unit provides the nicotine hit that smokers crave. It gives you the full effect of smoking real tobacco without harsh tobacco smoke and without the risk of fire. You have to charge up the cigarette, and there are cartridges to replace. There are many different brands online. For more information, call 1-866-997-2332.

> *"Rob authorized a neighbor to work on his car so he could get back on the road, running up over a thousand dollars in repairs before I realized what was going on. (He couldn't drive by this time.) The neighbor bought the car from us and sold it, giving us the difference."*

Insights: With a serious issue like keeping track of the patient's money, it may be necessary to get a power of attorney regarding financial matters. One of the first things that my mother did when she found out she had a serious illness was insist on going to the bank to make sure that I had control of her finances—in the likely event that she became unable at some point to do that. In the example, the neighbor was taking advantage of the patient, so if something like this happens to your loved one, you should discuss it with the person doing the work. Inform vendors and contractors that they should get approval from you before contracting any work—or they may not get paid. If power of attorney can't be obtained, make an effort to be part of the decisions regarding any major cash outlays. At least there was no car to worry about the patient driving. Things like this might pop up, but then plan what you need to do to prevent it from happening again.

Suspiciousness and paranoia.

Criticisms and accusations from the patient can be really hard to take. Relatives and friends of brain illness patients who are accused of stealing or lying can feel devastated. It's important to remember that you cannot convince your loved one that his or her suspicions are unfounded. Because of their inability to reason and impaired short-term memory, they may not be able to remember the explanation that you gave just minutes ago!

When your loved one makes accusations, try to remember that it's the disease speaking. Dealing with the situation comes down to you looking out for yourself.

If the accusation is directed at another person (Mable down the hall stole my purse, for example), first confirm that they aren't true in a diplomatic (not accusatory) way. After you find the purse safely tucked away, reassure the patient—don't agree with false accusations.

Here are some suggestions:

- If there are others that you're concerned about misunderstanding what's happening financially (siblings, for example), seek advice from a reputable third party. Try to arrange a family meeting.

- Maintain an up-to-date inventory of the patient's possessions.

- Whenever feasible, have the patient participate with financial matters, unless this creates more tension. Review the bills, and have him or her sign the checks.

- If the accusation stings, try to hold onto your temper. Leave the room or take a walk.

- Confide in someone that you trust to give you advice and help you cope.

- Acknowledge the emotions of fear and loss of control from the patient's viewpoint. Obviously, their independence is threatened, and that makes them lash out.

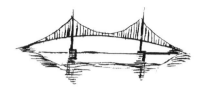

CHAPTER TWELVE

Irritability or Anger—
Look for the Stimulant!

WE ALL HAVE our limits. Under some circumstances, anger is understandable. In fact, it can be a necessary form of release. Among other causes, the brain cancer patient's anger may stem from pain, fear, and from a feeling of having no control over what is happening in their life. Be prepared, because the ones closest to the patient will often feel the sting of frustrated words. If they try to push you away, hold them tighter.

> *"Mom was angry at the cancer. She had lived a healthy life, and felt this was so unfair."*

Insights: One normal question among cancer victims is, "Why me?" Gordon asked that often. What unfortunate happenstance causes one person to have brain cancer and another not to have it? Sometimes he would ask, "Was I a bad person to have this happen to me?" The best medicine for your loved one is your sympathetic love and support. Make it known to them often through words and deeds, and reassure them that—whatever the cause of their cancer—it wasn't bad thoughts, stress, moral deficiencies, or character defects. It may help to let them know that you are an innocent bystander without any control of the situation either.

Gordon was very angry in the final weeks of his life, and he sometimes looked at me with a hateful glare. He treated his sisters with total courtesy, but I was often seen as the bad guy. I know that he loved me and would never have acted this way towards me under normal circumstances. Once I even asked him why he was looking at me like he hated me, and he denied it. Bitterness and resentment may mean that your loved one wants something from you that he or she isn't getting.

> *"Every now and then, Rob would give me such a look of hate. When I'd talk with him about it, he admitted that he was just so angry that this was happening. I never felt threatened by him. He was easily irritated, but extremely patient when it concerned Jack (his son)."*

Insights: Try to respond to the emotion behind the behavior. Validate the feelings, which are obviously strong. Realize that the anger is more with the situation than with any person. Wouldn't you be frustrated? Speak calmly and softly to the person. And now may not be the time to address your own feelings. The description was that the look was hateful, but it could have just as easily been a look of frustration. Help the patient understand what's happening within his or her own emotions. Don't call them on it, but work through the emotions with a counselor or chaplain. It isn't easy—for either the patient or the caregiver.

In all honesty, this is one situation where it's really hard to guard your heart, because you've already had it stomped on before you realize it. The action was unexpected and got caught up in another already exposed nerve. However, allowing our feelings to remain pummeled is our choice. And there was some jealousy involved—we were seeing the patient react differently to others in our presence. The patients themselves are most likely unaware of what they're exposing, and we should beware our own interpretation of what they're showing.

> *"My brother felt he was well enough to go home, and that was his entire focus the final six months of his life. Every day he wanted to leave. He lived on cigarettes and coffee, with little concern for reasonable meals."*

Insights: It's obvious why this bothered his family—this patient had lost his internal fight to live. Along with acceptance of his fate, he had decided to do it his way. But watching what they consider to be self-destructive behavior is hard for family members. What we see as "reasonable" wasn't what he saw as reasonable. In a situation like this, you could offer him other things he likes, which will make you feel better if he eats it, but choose your battles wisely. Unless there is still hope that he will survive, allow the patient to eat when and what he wants. I've heard of many people—including Gordon—living on ice cream in their final weeks of life. And let him smoke, as long as he doesn't burn anything down. It's not a health issue; it's a safety issue.

Wise words from Aristotle concerning anger:

"Anybody can become angry—that is easy; but to be angry with the right person, and to the right degree, and at the right time, and for the right purpose, and in the right way—that is not within everybody's power and is not easy."

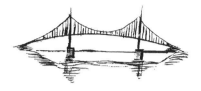

CHAPTER THIRTEEN

Indifference, Sadness, or Depression

B RAIN CANCER IS a serious and often debilitating illness. Depression can become a serious concern for the patient and everyone involved in his or her care. A depressed person may experience symptoms such as a profound loss of interest in normal activities, changes in appetite and sleep patterns. They can become restless, irritable, and agitated. If depression is not treated, it may become extreme. This can lead to a feeling of worthlessness, hopelessness, or extreme sadness.

> *"Bo, while never chatty, became withdrawn and quiet. He loved music, but no longer wanted to enjoy it. He was always strong and wanted to take care of me, but he did not even want to learn how to use the catheter. He asked me to do it for him. That wasn't like him."*

Insights: Lack of interest in something that they usually enjoy—such as music—is an indication of depression. Sit and talk with them to explore what's happening: "You seem down. Is something new happening for you? Is there anything that might make you feel better?" Try a different route if they won't open up to you. If you suspect that the patient is excessively anxious, talk to a doctor. Antidepressants can be helpful, but finding a way to offer encouragement will help, too. That's just not easy to do if the patient is dying. Explore what interests remain, and try to provide those activities for them—for example, read to them from their favorite book. Try to create moments of joy that you'll both cherish. Don't become discouraged if you're unable to find something right away. Keep trying.

> "He became sad towards the end of his life because he wanted to be able to spend more time with his immediate family members. He felt that some were not spending as much time with him as he wanted them to. He did not realize or would not admit to himself that they might be having a hard time dealing with his impending death and his plans to end his life."

Insights: Talk of suicide would be uncomfortable for anyone, especially those who love you. In a situation like this, you should discuss the problem with the patient, his family members, and friends. Explore ways to help others be more comfortable so that they'll continue to visit. Ask the patient to avoid sensitive topics when others are close by. If he or she seems unaware of what those topics are, offer to create a time-out signal—some word like "caterpillar," for example. When that word is spoken, a change in conversation is in order. Make sure it's odd enough so the message is clear. In addition to serving a purpose, creating a secret word will possibly add a little humor to an otherwise tense situation.

> "When Brian was told that he had a short time to live, we asked what arrangements he'd like in the way of burial, cremation, or a veteran's burial. He simply said he didn't care."

Insights: This reminds me of when I asked Gordon about where he wanted to be buried. We waited too long to have that discussion, too. Once you've broached the subject, don't take the initial "I don't care" as the final answer. Offer options and give suggestions. When you believe that the patient is having a day of clarity, take that opportunity for serious discussions. After a decision is made, try to clarify it later to be sure.

You also have to consider what other members of the family need for processing their grief. When my father died, he had made it clear that he wanted to be cremated, but his sister adamantly wanted a visitation with an open casket. We made both happen. You can and should consider the needs of others.

Author's note: Within two weeks of Gordon's death, I had my own personal will, living will, healthcare power of attorney—all pertinent death related documents and instructions—in legal form.

Wall of Inspiration—Two for One

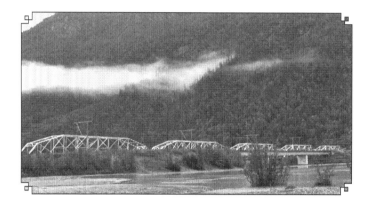

T HE NEUROSURGEON ON the other end of the phone wasn't what I expected. His patient was a high school math teacher, associate pastor, husband and father. Diagnosed with brain cancer, Mike and his wife were determined to fight. Coincidentally, another friend of Mike's—also an associate pastor—had that same type of brain cancer.

Mike was blessed to have a determined neurosurgeon and oncologist, who both believe in treating the physical and spiritual person. God was also part of his team—Mike knew it was in His hands, even though the prognosis was fourteen months. After surgery and months of chemotherapy, he was grateful to be alive.

Unfortunately, the tumor came back for a second round. Mike asked for a two-week grace period before surgery. The doctor was surprised, but he knew that it had to be important—and he believed that it wouldn't make any difference. After the surgery and recuperation, Mike called his neurosurgeon and said, "God told me to call you and tell you why I needed those two weeks." Being a man of faith, the doctor wasn't surprised. He was, however, amazed to hear how Mike spent his two-week reprieve. He had been surfing in California with his sixteen-year-old son. Surfing is a very physical sport, yet this brain cancer patient was able to go and enjoy that special time with his son.

Mike's friend the associate pastor died. He stood before those in attendance at his funeral and said, "I wouldn't change places with anyone here." He went on to say that his cancer had enlightened his life and affirmed his faith.

This amazing man is now a seventeen-month survivor—he's still alive. Unfortunately, so is the cancer. It's trying to make a third appearance.

What impressed me almost more than the story about the patient was the testimony of his neurosurgeon. He admitted that he keeps a personal inspirational journal about many of his patients. His chosen profession has to be tough, but it's obvious that he loves and respects God and the people they treat together.

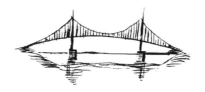

CHAPTER FOURTEEN

Concerns for the Caregiver

"The common bond of caregiving is the sense of isolation that comes from living outside the norm, from having everyday activities of life—dressing, walking, toileting, thinking clearly—that everyone else takes for granted, become such a big focus in your own life."

The Common Bonds of Caregiving by Suzanne Mintz

Neysa and I know firsthand that caring for a person with a brain illness is caregiving on a different level. It's not a matter of supplying basic needs. It's starting from scratch without knowing which direction will come close to working. Needs may change from moment to moment, and they may be more complex than you ever imagined. Simply put, you're caregiving in an environment that's not normal with tools that are designed to work within the normal scheme of things.

"It is important for the caregiver to have some time for themselves. Again, I didn't do this, and I spent every moment that I wasn't working with my husband. After a couple of years, this became very exhausting, and I'm sure my husband picked up on it. Toward the end, he said to me, 'Please don't be mad at me.' It made me realize that he saw my frustration and exhaustion, which wasn't fair to either of us."

Insights: As a brain cancer caregiver, usually the last thing that you want to think about is yourself. It's almost like you feel guilty—my husband, parent, sibling, child, or friend is critically ill, how can I think of myself? Here's how and why: If you get sick, the well-being of the patient *may be at risk.* Therefore food, rest, counseling, exercise, taking your medicine—all of those things that you do to keep yourself fit—are even more important.

There is a balance. Maintaining it in the worst days of your life can be an impossible dream. The very best that you can do is 1) focus on your health and sanity; and 2) focus on your loved one's health and sanity. Language allows us to make it sound so easy, but it's not.

> *"He would get frustrated if I was sad or upset about his cancer. His response would be to threaten to leave me because he felt I couldn't handle his illness and the prospect of his death."*

Insights: Sometimes the patient doesn't want to see emotion in the caregiver. It makes their situation too hard and too real. This is why friends have to be available for "consultation" 24/7. Emotions don't keep regular working hours, or even waking hours, and this may be the time the caregiver has to vent without upsetting the patient. Since those occasions are often unexpected, your friend will probably be alone—technically. Being a true friend means that you have your "available" sign on, no matter what time it is.

The Caregiver's Bill of Rights:

I have the right: To take care of myself. This is not an act of selfishness. It will enable me to take better care of my loved one.

I have the right: To seek help from others even though my loved one may object. I recognize the limits of my own endurance and strength.

I have the right: To maintain facets of my own life that do not include the person I care for, just as I would if he or she were healthy. I know that I do everything that I reasonably can for this person, and I have the right to do some things for myself.

I have the right: To get angry, be depressed, and express other difficult emotions occasionally.

I have the right: To reject any attempt by my loved one (either conscious or unconscious) to manipulate me through guilt, anger, or depression.

I have the right: To receive consideration, affection, forgiveness, and acceptance from my loved one for as long as I offer these qualities in return.

I have the right: To take pride in what I am accomplishing and to applaud the courage it sometimes takes to meet the needs of my loved one.

I have the right: To protect my individuality and my right to make a life for myself that will sustain me when my loved one no longer needs my full-time help.

From *Caregiving: Helping an Aging Loved One* by Jo Horne

I had been Gordon's primary caregiver through two unbelievably difficult years. When we brought him home with hospice, I wanted to spend every waking moment with him. I didn't know what moment would be his last, and I wanted to be there for him. The first week, the nurses told us he could die at any time. I was an emotional wreck. The second and third weeks, he rallied. By then I was a mental wreck from trying to keep up with the mental changes Gordon was going through; he was dragging me along. The fourth and fifth weeks were preambles to his death. By then, I was emotionally, mentally, and physically drained, and I had never been more unprepared to face Gordon's loss.

Perseverance comes with doing the very best that you can and realizing that you're human. Using the methodology in this book will get you closer to a peaceful existence when your loved one has brain cancer, but there has only been one perfect person, and He died for us. Prayer is important. Faith is important. Doing the very best you can and being left with minimal regrets and "if onlys" is worth all of the treasure in the world.

> *"As difficult as it is, you need to accept and try to deal with the reality of your situation. I lived in denial throughout my husband's illness, and because of that, I did not handle certain situations very well. For example, there were times that I went to work even though he was in very bad shape. I did not recognize this and felt that if I went to work, that meant that everything was okay. I wish I hadn't done that because I'm sure that made it harder on my husband."*

Insights: Acceptance is a process, composed of many small steps. The path to acceptance comes through facing each small loss as you go along, and allowing yourself time to grieve over each. If you're unable to break it down into smaller losses (such as the loss of companionship, physical closeness, social loss), then you aren't emotionally ready to accept what is happening and to just be with the person you love.

The caregiver in this example was experiencing unnecessary guilt; she did the best she could at the time. Some of us take longer to work through the losses because we're more comfortable staying with the idea that things are not going to change. Confronting that as soon as it's comfortable to do so will make the reality easier to deal with. Defiance prevents moving forward and causes you to be less capable of relating to the patient. Be kind with yourself; change isn't easy, and neither is grief.

I can't offer you any miracle advice to get through possibly the most difficult days of your life. What I can do, however, is offer you some insights to maintain your sanity. A very fine hospice chaplain named Ric Durham calls the following one-minute vacations.

When you need "feel good" senses.

Perhaps the song "My Favorite Things" said it best: "I simply remember my favorite things, and then I don't feel so bad." Start by writing down your five favorite sounds, smells, tastes, sights, and feels, putting them in a jar (Ric is from the mountains of North Carolina, so he recommends a Mason jar), and pulling them out one or two at a time on bad days. Savor each experience again in your mind. As the Julie Andrews song implies, it can push your mind back to a more positive place. Some examples:

Sounds: A kitten purring, a waterfall, a lullaby, bacon sizzling, a perfectly hit golf ball.

Feels: A baby's skin, a puppy's fur, silk, a rose petal, a velour blanket.

Here are some additional recommendations:

Try to be specific. For example, making snow cream after the second snow-fall of the season (which was rare when I was growing up in the South—not sure what was wrong with the first snow, but we always had to wait it out for the next snow). The smell of honeysuckle after a rainstorm. The scent and feel of a newborn baby. Let the memory take you away to a better frame of mind.

Sidestep memories that are beautiful, but painful. I love toasted marshmallow s'mores, but that reminds me too much of sitting around the campfire with Gordon enjoying that special treat. Sunrises and sunsets are beautiful, but if you've always shared them with your loved one, those memories may be too upsetting.

Keep a second jar to deposit your sad thoughts. Make it an exchange program—take out a pleasurable thought from one jar, and then drop in a painful thought in the other one. If the system works for good thoughts, it should also purge bad ones.

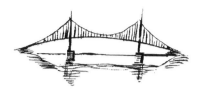

CHAPTER FIFTEEN

It's a "We" Thing—Impact on Family and Friends

WHAT YOU AND your loved one are going through has a direct impact on your family, friends, and community. Unless these other people are living with you, they may not know what you're experiencing. It's important that they do, so that they can help.

During most of our cancer battle, I know Gordon kept his sisters in the dark about his true condition. I, on the other hand, never sugar-coated the truth. So I seemed to be the one who cried wolf. Consequently, when he was in the hospital with the new diagnosis of metastatic brain cancer—especially as he was unable to communicate what was going on—I'm not sure what they thought. The important thing was that they came to us without question.

> *"When we first found out that he was terminally ill with brain cancer, my mother offered her sympathy and said, 'I have no idea what you must be going through.' Her honesty meant so much to me, and it is something I will always remember."*

Insights: Offer sympathy, not empathy. Don't say things like, "I know what you're going through," unless you've truly walked the exact same path.

Also stay away from statements like, "Everything is going to be alright." After the death of my father, nothing irked me more than that statement. Listening is sometimes the best gift that you can give to someone who is in a difficult life situation. A sympathetic shoulder to cry on is always in demand. It's easy, and it doesn't require a single spoken word!

> *"My family helped me the most by just being there for me when my husband and I needed help, whether it was emotional support or help with caring for him. His mom and sister also helped a lot by doing things with our son, and helping me clean up the house, do laundry, grocery shopping, etc. Being a caregiver takes a tremendous amount of energy, and since my husband could no longer work, I had to keep up with my full-time job in addition to caring for him."*

Insights: Support from family and friends is absolutely critical. Keeping all facets of life well balanced and keeping the balls from dropping can be an overwhelming effort. In this case, even simple things like helping around the house and spending time with the patient were invaluable. There may be needs due to changing family dynamics, especially if there are children or young adults involved. These age groups may never have experienced difficult and demanding life changes. Assistance may come in many different forms and functions—asking what help is needed is the most direct method.

Caregivers should always remember that the key to not being alone is letting people in. God will provide the support you need, if you will open up and accept it. Cherish those who give; forgive those who can't—some people feel very uncomfortable around any form of hardship. It's an unfortunate truth. Have faith that there will be enough willing hands to help you. And learn to ask for what you need.

> *"Rob's tumor returned with a vengeance after we had moved six hundred miles from our family, and only seven months after our son was born. Virginia only has in-home hospice and it's sporadic, so trying to work, raise our infant son, and care for a two-hundred-pound stubborn man with brain cancer—all with few friends and no family nearby—was nearly impossible."*

Insights: Difficult challenges never seem to happen at an opportune time or in an opportune place. When a family's normal support system is not around, the help may have to come from new friends, churches, and others in the community. It's amazing how many people truly want to help, if you'll only ask. Helping makes them feel better, and you will benefit greatly from their caring support.

Ways for friends to help:

1) Visiting can be a blessing or a curse. If you plan to visit, always call ahead. This will offer the caregiver an opportunity to give you an honest heads-up about what to expect, and a chance to schedule around their needs.

2) Skip the flowers and plants. First of all, they give the family one more thing to take care of. Secondly, they can give a funereal effect that the family doesn't need.

3) Cards, notes, banners, drawings—all heartfelt messages of love and support are appreciated. Don't just send them once; you can send them often throughout a cancer battle.

4) If you can, supply a meal or casserole approximately every three days, even if they say they don't need anything. If the family doesn't feel up to a visit, hand it to them when they open the door. However, never bring food if you're feeling under the weather.

5) Offer delivery food gift cards—pizza is a great pick-me-up. This will give the family a much-needed reprieve from cooking and a break from the cost.

6) Arrange for help with the laundry and housecleaning. You can arrange this with a local cleaning service, or get some friends together and schedule a day to go over and perform different tasks. Ask the family to make a job jar, and then come over every day or so and take care of a chore from it.

7) There will be other maintenance tasks that need to be done. Offer to cut the grass, trim the shrubs, or weed the flowerbeds. These are things that can slip through the cracks. If the front door squeaks, bring some oil.

8) Some people assume that the family wants time alone. This assumption can leave hurt feelings that can never be repaired. Short visits are sometimes a pleasant — and much needed — diversion. Don't procrastinate—just go.

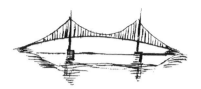

CHAPTER SIXTEEN

Understanding Anticipatory Grief

NTICIPATORY GRIEF REFERS to the difficult period before an impending loss. The patient who is dying can also experience it. The five stages of grief (denial, bargaining, depression, anger, and acceptance) will likely be present in the anticipatory grief process. Anxiety, dread, guilt, helplessness, hopelessness, and feeling overwhelmed are also very common.

Anticipatory grief is not simply grief before the actual loss. It may include a heightened concern for the dying person, rehearsal of the death, and even attempts to adjust to the consequences. This pre-loss period can allow people to resolve issues with the dying person and to say goodbye, although these might be more complicated if the loved one has brain cancer.

One obvious downside to anticipatory grief is witnessing your loved one's struggle with his or her impending death. As their condition worsens, you may grieve with each downturn and feel helpless. You may feel as if you are living with an empty pit in your stomach. It's normal for someone facing death to feel fear, pain, or anger. These feelings may be intensified with a loved one dying of brain cancer, where the emotions are already scrambled. This can be devastating to those seeking to shelter the patient. Hospice workers or counselors may be able to help.

> *"It is important to acknowledge that your loved one is going to die, so that you can find out their wishes, etc. I refused to accept that my husband was going to die, so he was not able to share his feelings with me (or anyone)."*

Insights: We often hear people say that grieving families who have known that a loss was coming had time to prepare. If the loved one and their family can form some kind of closure, then that does provide some relief. Anticipatory grief doesn't, however, take the place of post-loss grief. In fact, researchers suggest that to start to grieve as though the loss has already happened can leave the family feeling guilt for partially "abandoning" the patient or wishing that their suffering would end through their death. Painful topics that are staring you in the face—such as death, end of life wishes, and after-death preparation—are all hard to discuss.

Gordon and I had tactfully avoided the topic of death while we were fighting the hard battle to save his life. Therefore, I didn't even know where he wanted to be buried. His parents were buried in Michigan, but that would make it impossible for me to visit his grave very often. One particularly lucid day, I broached the subject. At first, he said he wanted to be buried close to where we liked to go on vacation. Over lunch, he informed me that he wanted to be buried with his Uncle Herb (who was next to his parents).

> *"I had to accept that I could fight all I wanted to, but the tumor was winning. The decision was made to take him back home to Michigan, where his family and friends could visit him, and he would have round-the-clock care. The day I took him back to Michigan remains the hardest day of my life."*

Insights: Anticipatory grief might actually be worse than real grief. It's what you feel when you're watching and expecting someone you love to die. Even though you don't want it to, your mind wanders to your life without the person who is dying. You'll hate it, but it's natural, and it's a part of your necessary acceptance. But the knowing doesn't make it any easier.

When a loved one is dying, every day seems like an eternity—good or bad. It's hard to see their pain, and it's hard to experience your own pain. You may be horror-stricken to find yourself wishing for the end. After I finally admitted this to the hospice chaplain, he asked me this question: "If you could do anything in the world to keep Gordon alive—with a good quality of life—would you do it?" Of course, the answer was yes.

"Most dying people—as well as their families and friends—go back and forth among the stages of dying, shifting from anger to denial to acceptance to bargaining to depression—many times, in no apparent order, and not necessarily in synchronization."

From *Final Gifts* by Maggie Callanan and Patricia Kelley

Hospice provides information on what to expect as your loved one goes through the dying process. There are times when the grief is so intense that you just can't stand it. It's okay to fall apart, but you can't fall so deeply that you can't get back up. Bouts of numbness can be a big relief. They do not mean you don't care.

"The most difficult aspect for me was the feeling of helplessness. I wanted so badly to help my husband through this difficult time in his life, and there was so little I could do to take away his pain and frustration. We both learned quickly that God is in control of our lives, and we all need to realize that."

Insights: We have a tendency to define "help" as being able to do something specific, while we are often most helpful by just being there and offering comfort.

≈

"God grant me the serenity to accept the things I cannot change."

Be patient, strong, and have peace within yourselves that once you do *everything you can*, you will be able through faith to accept the outcome. You don't have the ability to change the fact that your loved one has brain cancer or is dying. One of my mother's favorite statements is "God doesn't make mistakes." At times like these, that's a bitter pill to swallow.

"God grant me the courage to change the things I can."

Courage is many things, but I believe that this refers to the spirit of strength that enables us through faith to face our fears with confidence and resolution. A social worker once told me that having a loved one diagnosed with cancer is like being dropped in the middle of a deep jungle without any jungle training. While in that jungle, your survival skills would kick in, and you would fight with courage. When the care receiver has brain cancer, the jungle is even deeper and trickier to maneuver.

Use every tool that God has given you. Pray every prayer that will get you through, especially on those days where courage is hard to find.

"God grant me the wisdom to know the difference."

Wisdom is discretion and intuitive understanding. We develop it through trials and years. It's hard to find in times when sorrow is so deep that you are overwhelmed by it. Unfortunately, that's usually when you need wisdom the most. That's why we pray for that wisdom, that knowledge that we need. Past that mindset, do the very best that you can.

Closure

"Overall, despite how Mom's body failed, she did it with grace and above all humor. She called her cancer 'Mr. Icky,' her hand that no longer worked 'Petunia,' and her walker (which was outfitted with pink tennis balls) 'Trigger.' Every morning she would say a little prayer to her courage angel, raise her arms up in a V (or as close to it as she could), and say

'We Can Do It.' She was an amazing, beautiful, courageous, funny, unique woman, and I miss her every day."

Lack of Closure

"The most difficult aspect was not understanding how quickly he could be gone. He was absolutely fine one day, and then gone very fast. I had no time to say goodbye. Brian had fallen ill, {was} transferred from a nursing home to the emergency room, and I was told by the admitting nurse that he wasn't that bad. I asked if I should come down immediately, and she advised that I not overreact. I couldn't get the doctor to call me back. I took a plane from Denver to see him in the hospital in Florida. However, five minutes before I arrived, he had lapsed into a coma and never awoke. The difficult aspect is that things could have been different. I needed closure and was prevented from having it."

Hearing a story like this one makes me cringe. If your loved one is dying and you feel that the information you're being given is inaccurate, tell the person on the other side of the phone that you want to speak to their immediate supervisor *right now.* There is a time to practice courtesy and a time to make waves. (I should also note that this was not the first problem with this facility, so there was a foundation of mistrust.)

One of the biggest regrets that many people have after losing a loved one is that they failed to fully express their love and appreciation while they had time. Unless the patient makes it clear that they do not want loved ones to gush over them, friends and family members should take every opportunity to talk about their happy memories and let the dying person know that they had a positive impact on the lives of those around them. This is not the time, however, to rehash old arguments or engage in battles over hurt feelings. Most relationships have their ups and downs, so when time is short, highlighting the good times is in order.

While it's hard to do, know that—even with a brain illness—time can be a blessing. Many people die suddenly, leaving no time for expressions of love, no time for the saying of things previously left unsaid. While stress and anxiety are natural offshoots of knowing that a death is coming, this advance warning allows patients, as well as those in their inner circle, to fully express their feelings for one another. But be aware that with a brain illness, quality time may be more limited than it seems. Don't put off those expressions of love that are good for both you and your loved one.

≈

Fulfilling final wishes.

Like so many men, Gordon had loved cars from the time he was a small boy. Not only could he drive anything with wheels, prior to his illness he often drove thousands of miles every week. So it wasn't a big surprise that during one of his infrequent visits outside, he asked, "Do you think we could go for a ride somewhere?" He was in a wheelchair and needed help to get him into and out of a vehicle, so we couldn't do it right then. Later it dawned on me—he might enjoy going for a ride in a utility truck instead of a car. He had sold them and loved them through his work. So I asked two of his friends to bring a small bucket truck and take him for a ride.

Everything was arranged. It took a while to get Gordon into the truck and ready to go. We thought it would be a long ride, but fifteen minutes later, they were back. I was a little hurt, but Gordon had gotten tired. Seeing the tears in his eyes told me what it had meant to him and to the guys who helped us out that day. Gordon thanked me over and over again. No one who was there that day will ever forget it as long as they live. Final gifts don't have to be outlandish—they just have to be important to your loved one.

Here are some other accounts of final wishes:

> *"Bo loved being outside and sometimes we would even sleep in our yard to enjoy the fresh air and stars. I took him outside in his wheelchair, spread a blanket, and lifted him down so that we could sit on the grass, and he just kept asking when we were going inside."*

> *"My mother was diagnosed with cancer when she was only fifty. Even though she was extremely ill the spring before she died, she insisted on taking my family to Disney World. It was a bittersweet trip. She was so brave and determined to enjoy being with her grandchildren, but she was so weak and fragile I feared for her safety. She finally relented and used a wheelchair, but when we got to the Swiss Family Robinson tree house, she parked the chair and climbed through it with her grandchildren, which was nothing short of a miracle!"*

When your loved one expresses a desire for a final wish, do whatever you can to make it happen. There may be concerns that come up because of their illness, but don't feel disappointed if they can only enjoy the experience for a short period of time. You did your part and fulfilled the wish.

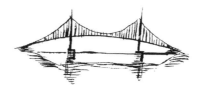

CHAPTER SEVENTEEN

Dealing with Difficult End-of-Life Topics

A S I'VE NEVER personally stared death in the face (except through Gordon's eyes), I can't speak firsthand of the powerful emotions that must be behind every terminal diagnosis. I did, however, have a conversation last night with a man who was in a horrible car crash and died two times. He remembers remarkable beauty and peace. His work on earth wasn't done, so Chris is still here. Talking with him reassures me about what I already know—death isn't the end. Whatever your beliefs, when you or someone you love is dying, the days ahead hold many impossible moments that only the greatest courage and much prayer can get you through—and the hope that you will be reunited in the future.

"The Elephant in the Room" by Terry Kettering
There's an elephant in the room.
It is large and squatting,
so it is hard to get around it.

Yet we squeeze by with,
"How are you?" and "I'm fine,"
and a thousand other forms of trivial chatter.

We talk about the weather.
We talk about work.
We talk about everything else,
except the elephant in the room.

There's an elephant in the room.
We all know it's there.
We are thinking about the elephant
as we talk together.

It is constantly on our minds.
For, you see, it is a very big elephant.
It has hurt us all, but we do not talk about
the elephant in the room.

≈

> *"The only time I saw my husband's fear was a few weeks before he passed away when the doctors told us there was nothing more they could do for him. He was in the hospital at the time and thought his death was imminent. I reassured him that the doctors said he still had weeks to live. Although that in itself was a scary thought, when you think you are literally about to die, weeks sound like a gift."*

Insights: It is important to reassure your loved one that they will not be alone, and that you will remain with them even after death. Often, a person needs to know that he or she has done all they could within their life. This is a universal human concern. Reassure your loved one that you will do everything in your power to make sure that they will not hurt. There may be pain in the period leading up to death, but healthcare providers and hospice nurses will do what is necessary to keep them comfortable as they die. Death itself will not hurt. After death, the pain will never return.

"A dying person's depression grows out of grief. Dying people grieve as anyone does for something that is lost. But their grief has two parts; they're mourning what's lost already to illness—health, family role, job, independence—but also for what will be lost when they die—personal relationships, life itself, and the future. These feelings of sadness and depression should be honored, not dismissed or diluted."

From *Final Gifts* by Maggie Callanan and Patricia Kelley

I read an article about an eighty-six-year-old man with stage IV abdominal cancer. It said that the man isn't worried about death itself. He is at peace with dying, and he has no regrets—in fact he has already had the marker put on his cemetery plot. It's the pain he worries about. "Death itself is not a fearful consideration for me," he said. "But the process of dying could be if it were excruciatingly uncomfortable."

Though he's not in any hurry to die, he anticipates that he will feel severe pain when the cancer reaches its final phases, and when that happens, he wants a doctor to be able to prescribe him a lethal dose of medication that he can use to end his life peacefully. "I don't think of it as suicide because I'm dying anyway," he said.

Final Gifts is a peaceful book on death and dying, and I recommend that everyone read it. It was written by several hospice nurses to document many wonderful accounts of people dying peacefully and even happily. Many had cancer. Reading that book convinced me—once and for all—that death doesn't have to be the horrible experience that we so often see dramatized on television or in movies. If we expedite death unnaturally, we may well be depriving ourselves of giving and receiving gifts of love.

Since I'm not dying (that I know of), I don't know how I'd feel. But I can offer you this through faith—I have seen enough to make me realize that there are worse things than death itself. And I can promise you that Gordon's death wasn't peaceful, but it wasn't nightmarish either. I attribute that in some ways to his brain cancer. I don't think that he was ever able to achieve serenity because of the turmoil going on in his brain.

"'Dying is always painful.' This is one of the most common misconceptions about dying. Pain can be relieved safely without any danger of death or addiction. Hospice caregivers and most doctors are familiar with the proper use of analgesic drugs. When given in the correct dose at the right time, pain can be relieved without sedating the patient. When pain is relieved, patients can experience a good quality of life until the time that death occurs. Good pain management does not shorten the course of life. On the contrary, patients who receive excellent pain management tend to live longer than expected."

From "Myths about Dying" on the Hospice Foundation of America Web site

≈

Consider these reasons that we might fear death:

We fear the unknown sting of death. We don't view it as a fulfillment of a journey well lived. We fear the unknown. We fear the pain that may accompany death.

We don't want to leave the ones that we love. It has taken a while, but I've come to the realization that our loved ones really don't leave us. Oh, I'm not talking about ghosts. I'm talking about the memories left behind and their presence in our lives. *They are always close.*

We fear what will happen to our loved ones after we die. I attended the saddest funeral. It was a simple graveside service. As the service began, the middle-aged widow sat alone on the front seat facing the open grave. I was shocked! Before the service, the funeral director asked that others step up in place of family. Thank God they did—what an awful thought to sit alone on the worst day of your life!

We're not ready to meet our God. When a brain illness occurs, we need to do everything that we can to prepare our loved one for the meeting, and trust that God will take care of the rest.

So what realization would have helped comfort me the most when Gordon died? God can restore whatever cancer (or any other illness) takes away. This is our final and greatest gift from our Creator.

> *"At my mother's funeral I asked the minister to read the following short segment that was special to her from Robert Fulghum's book,* All I Ever Needed to Know I Learned in Kindergarten:
>
> *I believe that imagination is stronger than knowledge.*
> *That dreams are more powerful than facts.*
> *That hope always triumphs over experience.*
> *That laughter is the only cure for grief.*
> *And I believe that love is stronger than death."*

Seeing people who aren't in the room—or are they?

> *"This happened toward the end of my husband's life. I wasn't sure at the time if he was transitioning to the next world, but he would talk about people who weren't in the room. I simply went along with what he was saying for fear of confusing him even more."*

You can believe what you want—or at least whatever your faith and experiences dictate—but for myself, I prefer to believe that death is a reuniting with loved ones who have gone before us through the death portal. Who knows what her husband saw, but the visions didn't seem to disturb or concern him. Was it the brain cancer?

"The experience of dying frequently includes glimpses of another world and those waiting in it. Although they provide few details, dying people speak with awe and wonder of the peace and beauty they see in this other place. They tell of talking with, or sensing the presence of, people whom we cannot see—perhaps people they have known and loved."

From *Final Gifts* by Maggie Callanan and Patricia Kelley

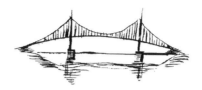

CHAPTER EIGHTEEN
More Than Just Difficult Thoughts of Death

The hospice motto: Live fully until you die.

L AST EVENING WHILE we were out having a glass of wine and listening to music, we met another couple doing the same. The woman and I chatted, and she asked me what I do for a living. I told her that I write books on cancer and grief. Instantly, her look turned hard. She told me that her sister had died just the week before after the breast cancer she had battled for ten years went to her brain. But there was more...she told me that if I would write a book on assisted suicide she would buy it. Had her sister voiced that desire before the brain cancer? I don't know; some considerations transcend our human ability to process. There was much bitterness in her sister. I had ruined her night of trying to forget, so we moved on. She'll have to fight her demons on her own terms, just as I did with Gordon. And next time I'm asked what I do for a living in a bar, I may just say something like, "I'm a podiatrist."

When we talk about suicide and assisted suicide in a terminal cancer patient, these topics shake our moral belief foundation. My personal concern is this—I've seen a lot of "terminal" cancer patients walking around many years after their death sentence. If we talk suicide or assisted suicide in a terminal cancer patient with brain cancer, my concern becomes wrapped around three words: "of sound mind." Ethically, I'd have to recuse myself either way, because I believe that though the last weeks with Gordon were torturous, in retrospect there was a reason for them.

Author's note: Before you read this chapter, I want to warn you in advance that one of the loved ones of a respondent did commit suicide. I feel it's an important message, so I'm leaving that story intact.

With death looming in the near future, Gordon asked me to use his medications to overdose him and end his life. My reply was simply, "Honey, I can't do that." He then asked, "Why not?" I didn't know what to say. Frankly, the real answer was that I couldn't have done it. No matter how much I loved him, I couldn't have done it. And in fact, I still believed—even with the turbulent times we were going through—that we could provide him with a somewhat peaceful passing. Some of that was selfish because I was still looking for my own closure. I was hoping for some touching and memorable moments to carry me through the upcoming years ahead without one of the cornerstones of my life.

We live in a society with a stigma about suicide. We are taught that it is not acceptable, both ethically and spiritually. But what if you are already dying? What if you fear the unknown of a death not on your own terms? Consequently, the final events and waiting for them might scare you so much that you want to stop the waiting. Neysa says that some people want to die, but don't want to be dead. There is much confusion in that thought, but it's sound logic. When you throw constant pain on top of that—well, it may not have been the confused reasoning of his brain illness that resulted in Gordon asking me to help him die. It's natural to think about the final moments of life and wonder if we can handle it. But hastening death is a heavy solution—one that those of us remaining on earth would have to live with.

In our case, determining what Gordon thought was intolerable was a much better solution. Was it really the pain, or did it just take too much energy to keep functioning? I should have asked, "Can you tell me what's bothering you that much?" I was afraid of the answer, but I could have perhaps given him some peace. If a similar discussion happens to you, reassure your loved one, and then explain what you will or won't do to make that happen. Let them know that—regardless of your love for them—you can't do anything to expedite their passing, but you'll be beside them and you'll help them in any way possible to live their last days peacefully.

> *"He would discuss his plans for ending his own life with his teenage son and discuss his plans in casual conversation with anyone he spoke with about his cancer, as if he were discussing plans for retirement."*

Insights: There are several disturbing aspects to this, including the patient's own feelings, the impact on the person who is telling about the experience, and—last but not least—the realization of what the teenage son must have felt hearing his father discuss suicide. In this case, the patient had repeatedly made it clear to his fiancée, son, and family that he had every intention of ending his life. In fact, these discussions with family members resulted in their staying away instead of giving their strong support to a dying man. The discussion itself may have been because he didn't want the people he loved to be surprised. Perhaps he wanted his loved ones and friends to understand so that the death act didn't seem like a rejection by him, or perhaps he was hoping to help them avoid the "blame stigma" of suicide. Or maybe it was just to see the son's response—do you care enough about me to talk me out of it? However, that doesn't seem to be the case in this situation.

Suicide—besides other emotional concerns—leaves a lack of closure for family and friends that can never be resolved. I know several widows of suicide victims who have convinced me of the long-term impact. The son will undoubtedly need counseling—if for no other reason than he might believe (after hearing this from his father) that suicide is acceptable behavior. That could be from a qualified counselor or hospice chaplain, if the son accepts their guidance. Support can come from peers, too.

Note to readers: This patient did commit suicide. Here is what his fiancée said: "My fiancé chose to shoot himself in the head. He made it quite clear *from the time of his diagnosis* that he would end his life on his terms. Those close to him—family and friends—were aware of his plans from that point, including his intended method. There was no talking him out of it. His decision (as he explained it) came from his belief in reincarnation and his desire not to suffer or be a burden to those who loved him. He needed to be in control of his life and his death."

Neysa's thoughts: The fiancée really did all she could do. She listened to him and his reasoning. She let him know her feelings and her love for him, and she made him aware of the impact on her and his family. That did not cause him to change his mind. I'm sure she would have explored with him the options besides suicide that would avoid the suffering that he feared, but that was not convincing to him. The fear of becoming a burden to your loved ones—coupled with the fear of a loss of independence and control—is something almost everyone struggles with over time. I'm sure she encouraged him to talk over his decision with anyone else who might be helpful, such as a counselor, a clergyperson, or his physician. The last thing she did was to recognize that she had done all that she could to dissuade him. That is obvious by her response after his death; she was not left with the grief issue of false guilt that she should have been able to prevent it. You do what you can as compassionately as you can, but you can't control what someone will choose to do.

(Note: As Neysa is a trained counselor, I wanted her to address this issue. She discussed her response with an ethicist, and he concurred.)

Several factors, such as uncontrolled pain, advanced illness, loss of control, and hopelessness, have been suggested as indicators for vulnerability to suicide in cancer patients. Patients with cancer do commit suicide more often than people without cancer; however, the numbers are very low. They are usually focused on *trying to live,* although metastatic growth and reoccurrence can throw them into depression.

Another area of concern is the fear of being a burden on others as the cancer progresses. In some cases this can be reframed into a realization that allowing others to care for you is a gift, through helping the patient to trust those who love him or her. It is important in all illness situations to protect the person's dignity to the end, and allow them as much independence, control, and decision-making power as possible.

Take all discussions of suicide seriously. In Gordon's case, I knew he wasn't serious. He had fought too hard to live. Now, that doesn't mean that I would have put a loaded gun in his hand. So why did he ask? If you can find the cause and address it, perhaps you can save a loved one from going to the extreme.

Also remember to secure the environment. Make sure there's no loaded gun in the nightstand. No knives within reach. No matches or lighters to threaten the safety of the patient or others. Keep strong drugs in a safe, unavailable place. These are things that you can do—but there is much that you can't. Work within the boundaries of what is realistic.

"Thinking of suicide, when it occurs, is frightening for the individual, for the healthcare worker, and for the family. Suicidal statements may range from an off-hand comment resulting from frustration or disgust with a treatment course, such as, 'If I have to have one more bone marrow aspiration this year, I'll jump out the window,' to a statement indicating deep despair and an emergency situation, such as, 'I can't stand what this disease is doing to all of us, and I am going to kill myself.' Exploring the seriousness of these thoughts is important. If the thoughts of suicide seem to be serious, then the patient should be referred to a psychiatrist or psychologist, and the safety of the patient should be secured."

From the National Cancer Institute Web site

The **QPR** suicide prevention model (question, persuade, refer) is patterned after the success of the **CPR** medical intervention and is based upon the following concepts:

1) Those who most need help in a suicidal crisis are the least likely to ask for it;

2) The person most likely to prevent a suicide is someone they already know; and

3) Prior to making a suicide attempt, a person typically sends warning signs.

Question the person about their suicide intentions.

Persuade the person that the days remaining are worth living.

Refer them for help to a chaplain, doctor, social worker, or hospice worker.

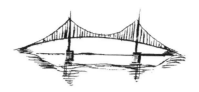

CHAPTER NINETEEN

Dealing with "What Ifs" and "If Onlys"

W<small>E PUT OUR</small> blinders on because the truth scares us so much we don't want to see it or believe it. People have off days, especially when stress and pain are daily companions. We know that what we're going through will change our world so catastrophically that we look away from the future.

In some ways, there are no more powerful words when used together than "what if" or "if only." Both imply regret and a desire to go back and take a different path.

So we need a plan to get rid of the "if only" and "what if" brain torture. Here is what I want you to do:

➢ Take out a blank sheet of paper. At the top, the header should read, "My If Only List."

➢ Begin to make a comprehensive list of all of your "if only" regrets. Take your time and be thorough. There is no "if only" too big and no "if only" too small for this list. They are all pertinent.

➢ After you have completed the first draft of the list, leave it and go do something else. Once you're away from the list for a while, other "if only" thoughts will surface that will need to be added.

➤ When your list is complete, I want you to hold it facing upward with both of your hands towards the sky and pray this prayer: "Lord, here are my 'if only' burdens. They are abusing my mind, heart, thoughts, and spirit. I know that they are not good for me. Please take them into your care. Thank you. Amen."

➤ After you have prayed, open your mind and imagine God's hand coming down from the clouds of heaven and taking all of the "if only" burdens off of that piece of paper. As far as you are concerned, the page is now empty.

➤ Take the "empty" piece of paper, tear it up into little pieces, and dispose of it with fervor. There are many ways of doing this: Throw the (biodegradable) pieces into the ocean. Flush them down the toilet. Bury them in a deep hole in the back yard and then plant a nice gardenia over them. Make it a ceremony. Play rock music or Beethoven's "Moonlight" Sonata. Celebrate the fact that your "if only" burdens are now in a much better place.

➤ This process may take several applications before you are rid of all "if only" or "what if" thoughts. Finally, they will no longer be a burden to you. They now belong to God. Be sure to thank him for taking them away and relieving your mind.

Believe me, I know that it is not always this simple. You can control your conscious thoughts, but not your subconscious. If you're a very patient believer, over time your reassurance will blossom like a new spring, and you will realize that those "if only" statements were preventing you from moving on with the rest of your life. They were holding you back and therefore were unhealthy. Now they are just where they need to be—on God's capable shoulders.

As you go through the intense process of healing, remember that the deepest wounds will fester and spread if left exposed and untreated. It's important to close them, and allow yourself to move forward. Scars are something that we all have on the inside and outside, but scars don't lead to a painful and senseless infection of our spirit.

"There is something beautiful about all scars of whatever nature. A scar means the hurt is over, the wound is closed and healed, done with."

Harry Crews

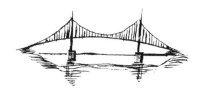

CHAPTER TWENTY

Finding Your Beacon Through the Storm Called "Grief"

Letter Twelve from *The Losing of Gordon: A Beacon Through the Storm Called "Grief"*

My dearest Gordon,

In the final weeks of your life, I knew that I would eventually need either counseling or exorcism—whichever came first. Those were very bad days and weeks. No offense, honey, but you were awfully hard on me. I recently met a man who had been through a severe brain trauma. He was trying to explain to me how you felt and what was possibly going through your mind during those final days. I can only hope that you are at peace now. Somehow, I have to move past that; but it's hard to rationalize. We loved each other so much, but love and hate is a fine line, and I think that in some ways you hated me in your final days. It's not going to be easy to get past that.

So, back to the subject of counseling—do you remember Pat at the cancer center? She and I were always close, so I've started going to her. Unfortunately, you know how stubborn I am. The first thing that I told her was that I wanted to know exactly when I would feel better…period. Can you imagine how irked I was when she told me that grief was a process? I don't like it. It hurts. I want it to go away. She said that out of respect for you, I needed to grieve. I love and respect her, but what? Like I could stop the grief from coming. Anyway, I will be going to her for a while. At least through the grief p-r-o-c-e-s-s.

By the way, I've just recently found out that those antidepressants that I had you taking to help during your cancer battle don't really work at all. At least the ones I've tried haven't. All they've done is cause bad side effects. Gloria has asked me to go back to the gym with her. Maybe I'll try that. It couldn't hurt my already low self-esteem. Evidently, my confidence in myself was buried along with you.

I miss you so much.

Love,
Joni

FAITH—Whether it washes over you like a gentle tide or engulfs you like a powerful wave, faith flows from your connection to God.

Joni James Aldrich

Grief insight #1: If the worst has happened, turn your caregiving *inward*, and remember that your loved one would want you to rebuild and go on. Others may help, but you alone can find your beacon through the storm called "Grief."

Grief insight #2: Turn towards your family, old friends, new friends, and your own inner spirit as you move forward.

Grief insight #3: God is not the enemy that you might believe in your pain. It took much to rebound my faith—there was some combination of four books (so far), two church families, long walks on the beach, homeopathic healers, strong goals, and much self-centering to get me past my rift with God. He must have thought, "How pigheaded can one person be?" But God—thankfully—is a patient and loving Savior.

Grief insight #4: Counseling is not for the weak, but for the strong. We have a stigma in our society that going to a "shrink" means you are mentally unstable. Personally, I think there is nothing unstable about knowing that you need help to sort out things that have rocked your world that are hard to deal with. Through the last awful weeks of Gordon's life, I always knew that I was going to need some help. Yet I look back at my first visit with my counselor Pat with much amusement. After I left I thought, "That didn't help at all." Yet, through the weeks that followed, Pat's words followed me everywhere.

Grief insight #5: You have to be open to the healing. Realize your pitfalls, and challenge them head-on. Accentuate your strengths, and let them take the forefront of your life. Above all else, do not curl up and wither away. You are still alive.

"The beach was swept away by the twin forces of violent wind and waves. Days later, piles of broken shells were deposited onto the shore. Nature had begun the rebuilding process. This is much the same as the process we undergo when rebuilding our lives after suffering the catastrophic loss of someone we love."

—Joni James Aldrich

Release your feelings here:

Today's feeling is (circle one) a happy blessing or a released burden:

_____

_____

_____

_____

_____

Today's feeling is (circle one) a happy blessing or a released burden:

_____

_____

_____

_____

_____

Today's feeling is (circle one) a happy blessing or a released burden:

_____

_____

_____

_____

_____

Today's feeling is (circle one) a happy blessing or a released burden:

_____

_____

_____

_____

_____

Today's feeling is (circle one) a happy blessing or a released burden:

_____

_____

_____

_____

_____

_____

Today's feeling is (circle one) a happy blessing or a released burden:

_____

_____

_____

_____

_____

_____

Today's feeling is (circle one) a happy blessing or a released burden:

_____

_____

_____

_____

_____

_____

Today's feeling is (circle one) a happy blessing or a released burden:

_____

_____

_____

_____

_____

_____

Today's feeling is (circle one) a happy blessing or a released burden:

_____
_____
_____
_____
_____
_____

Today's feeling is (circle one) a happy blessing or a released burden:

_____
_____
_____
_____
_____
_____

Today's feeling is (circle one) a happy blessing or a released burden:

_____
_____
_____
_____
_____
_____

Today's feeling is (circle one) a happy blessing or a released burden:

_____
_____
_____
_____
_____
_____

Today's feeling is (circle one) a happy blessing or a released burden:

_____
_____
_____
_____
_____
_____

Today's feeling is (circle one) a happy blessing or a released burden:

_____
_____
_____
_____
_____

Today's feeling is (circle one) a happy blessing or a released burden:

_____
_____
_____
_____
_____

Today's feeling is (circle one) a happy blessing or a released burden:

_____
_____
_____
_____
_____

RESOURCES:

American Cancer Society, 1-800-ACS-2345, www.cancer.org
American Society of Clinical Oncology, 1-888-651-3038, www.cancer.net
National Cancer Institute, 1-800-4-CANCER, www.cancer.gov
www.braintumor.org
www.nabraintumor.org
www.theibta.org
www.BrainTumorConnections.com
www.braintrust.org
www.twosistersonamission.com
www.karmanos.org
www.gildasclub.org
www.angelahospice.org
www.PeopleLivingWithCancer.org
www.braininjurymn.org
www.cancer.duke.edu/btc

Other books by author and speaker Joni James Aldrich

The Saving of Gordon: Lifelines to W-I-N Against Cancer

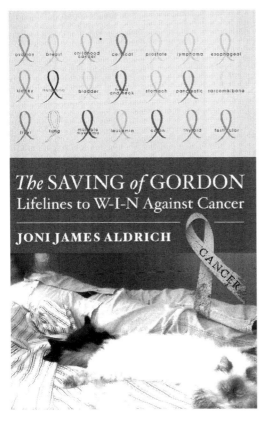

Cancer is the toughest fight many of us will ever face. Knowledge is your armor, and the right cancer treatment is your weapon. Two of this book's pivotal chapters will discuss the W-I-N method of finding the right cancer treatment facility and oncology team. Whether your cancer is a "cash cow" or rare, it's not about "simple"—it's about effective. Preparing for this battle will be a significant investment of your time, and it may mean leaving your comfort zone—so a well-formulated battle plan is a must. This book doesn't pretend to have all of the answers, but it does help you get your hands around the questions. Joni Aldrich has written a practical, powerful and movingly written companion that will guide patients and those who love them through the most arduous journey they'll ever face.

The Cancer Patient W-I-N Book: Our Cancer Fight Journal

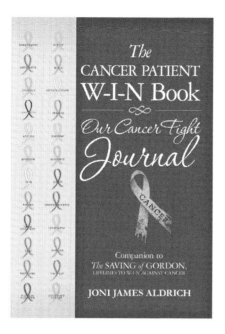

Utilizing the experience she gained as a cancer caregiver for her husband Gordon, Joni has created this useful workbook to document thirty-three of your oncologist visits. It incorporates many of the basic principles from *The Saving of Gordon,* and can help you stay focused and organized.

The Losing of Gordon: A Beacon Through the Storm Called "Grief"

If you should lose your battle to save your loved one's life, *The Losing of Gordon* provides a beacon of hope for those who are mourning. It is written around a series of letters that Joni wrote to her husband, Gordon, during her grief "process." Some are heartbreaking. Some are almost humorous lessons in perseverance. All are inspirational.

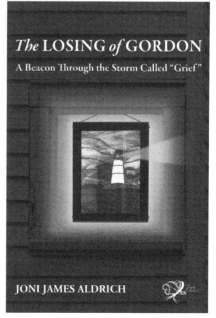

Index

Made in the USA
Lexington, KY
13 August 2014